The Complete Guide to Refractive Surgery

Stanley C. Grandon, M.D.

with Susan Giffin

PATTON PUBLISHING COMPANY
DEARBORN, MICHIGAN

THE COMPLETE GUIDE TO REFRACTIVE SURGERY
Copyright ©1999 by Stanley C. Grandon, M.D. and Susan Giffin. All rights reserved. Printed in the United States of America. No part of this book may be used or reproduced in any manner whatsoever without written permission except in the case of brief quotations embodied in critical articles or reviews. For more information, address

>Dr. Stanley C. Grandon
>Patton Publishing Company
>15212 Michigan Avenue
>Dearborn, Michigan 48126
>(313) 582-8856

or contact e-mail address:

>thewritestuff@visitus.net

Cover Design by Nicolas H. Khoury and Steve E. Ghannam

Text Design by IRIS Design & Print, Detroit, Michigan

Printing by Edwards Brothers, Ann Arbor, Michigan

THE COMPLETE GUIDE TO REFRACTIVE SURGERY is an expanded edition of GOOD-BYE, GLASSES, written by Susan Abbas [nee Giffin], published in 1990, and of the 1995 edition of THE COMPLETE GUIDE TO REFRACTIVE SURGERY, by Stanley C. Grandon, M.D., and Susan Giffin.

To all refractive surgery patients worldwide who, in their quest for better vision, have contributed significantly to the advancement of ophthalmic microsurgery

Acknowledgments

I wish to acknowledge the following people for their significant contributions to *The Complete Guide to Refractive Surgery*, directly or indirectly.

Professor Svyatoslav Fyodorov, Director of the Moscow Scientific Research Laboratory of Experimental and Clinical Problems of Eye Surgery, whose radial keratotomy (RK) procedure has revolutionized ophthalmology worldwide;

Leo D. Bores, M.D., Director of the Bores Eye Institute in Scottsdale, Arizona, without whose vision to bring RK to the United States, this book probably would not have been written;

Antonio Mendez, M.D., Mexico, who originated hexagonal keratotomy, the microsurgical procedure for correcting farsightedness;

Luis Ruiz, M.D., Mexico, who developed the surgical technique for correcting astigmatism, with or without other refractive surgery;

José Ignacio Barraquer, M.D., Colombia, who developed keratomileusis, the forerunner of today's LASIK surgery;

Gary M. Grandon, Ph. D., Associate Vice Chancellor for Computing and Imaging Systems at the University of North Carolina (Greensboro), whose computer wizardry enabled him to develop the computer software, which I have used successfully in my own practice, and who wrote Chapter 19 of this book;

Alan Spigelman, M.D., Michigan, who contributed a section on the Excimer Laser for Chapter 14, and also Chapter 15 on LASIK for myopia;

Henry Hirschman, M.D., New York, author of Chapter 17, for lending his expertise on intraocular lens implants, particularly for use in correcting high myopia and hyperopia;

Dennis Williams, M.D., Florida, author of Chapter 18 on clear lens implant, who has performed more secondary intraocular lens implants than any other eye surgeon in the United States;

Susan Giffin, who, with expertise in writing for the consumer, has painstakingly guided the development of this revised and expanded edition of her own *Good-Bye, Glasses*, the first consumer's guide to radial keratotomy and for which she traveled to Moscow, USSR, to personally interview Professor S. Fyodorov, the father of radial keratotomy. She also extensively interviewed Dr. Leo Bores, who brought RK to the United States.

Special thanks also to:

The staff of the Eye Surgery Institute of Dearborn, especially Frank R. Markey, M.D., and Michael Bialik, M.D. (both retired), who brought me into the practice many years ago; Thomas Borland, M.D., Ruth Boyman, M.D., Diana Zdun Jacobs, Marie McKeough, Marianne Ossenmacher, Barbara Johnson, Carol Scalici, Angela Babosh, and Debra Root who have worked with me for many years.

And, on a more personal note, my sincere appreciation to:

My wife, Barbara, and my three sons, Jeremy, Jonathan, and Peter, for their daily inspiration.

Last, but not least, I would like to acknowledge the thousands of surgery patients whose vision I have corrected over the years. In many respects, they are the true pioneers of ophthalmology.

Table of Contents

Foreword
Preface
Introduction

1. Anatomy of the Eye 1
2. The Eye Care Specialists 5
3. Myopia - Focusing on the Problem 9
4. Hyperopia and Astigmatism 15
5. Non-Surgical Treatments 21
6. RK - A Surgical Solution, Soviet-Style 31
7. RK - American Refinements 37
8. HK and AK - Mexican Developments, American Refinements 45
9. Criteria for Candidacy 55
10. Informed Consent – Making an Educated Decision 61
11. Refractive Surgery – The Operations 71
12. Post-Op Complications, Care, and Expectations 79
13. The Blue Cross Blues 85
14. Looking to Lasers – The Excimer and Holmium Lasers 91
15. LASIK 105
16. Hyperopic LASIK 117
17. Phakic IOL 121
18. Clear Lens Implants 125
19. Computers in Refractive Surgery 129
20. Patient Profiles 143
21. Questions & Answers 151
22. Summary 163

Glossary
Index

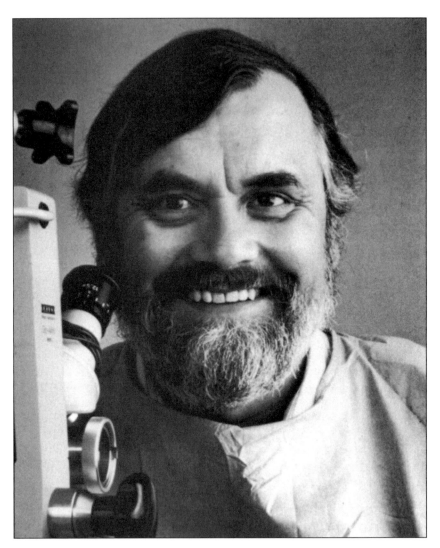
Leo D. Bores, M.D.

Foreword

Some 20 years ago, in an effort to learn more about intraocular lens implant techniques, I traveled to Russia and got sidetracked. As the saying goes, the rest is history…and therein lies a tale, one that has not been completely told to date.

The Complete Guide To Refractive Surgery makes a pretty good stab at it. In addition, it is one of the better works describing radial keratotomy from the patient's point of view. I recommend it to the lay reader for that purpose, and also to answer some inevitable questions.

The Complete Guide to Refractive Surgery is also recommended to the professional reader for the insights gained, not only into how the whole thing started but also into the mind of an individual who sets out to have his vision corrected.

I am sure that each class of reader will enjoy *The Complete Guide to Refractive Surgery.*

Leo D. Bores, M.D.

Preface

As an ophthalmologist who specializes in refractive surgery, I have always been keenly interested in new surgical techniques, treatments, and procedures that could impact my specialty.

When I attended medical school, there was no talk of surgical solutions to refractive errors. Eyeglasses and contact lenses were the accepted methods of correcting nearsightedness, farsightedness, and astigmatism.

Then, in the late 1970s, radial keratotomy (RK) captured my attention when Dr. Leo Bores performed the first RK operation in the United States at the Detroit Medical Center. I was fortunate to have assisted him on some of the early cases that followed.

Immediately after those introductory procedures, I refrained from performing RK on my own patients, primarily because I knew that significant refinements were needed before RK could become an accepted, established procedure in American ophthalmology.

The subsequent development of the diamond knife, the ultrasound pachymeter, and some of my own surgical instruments advanced the procedure significantly. In 1981, I began performing RK surgery on my own patients, and since then have performed more than 16,000 refractive surgeries of all types.

Likewise, in the late 1980s, I closely studied the work of Dr. Antonio Mendez of Mexico, who originated a procedure to correct farsightedness. After making certain modifications to his procedure, in 1991, I began performing hexagonal keratotomy (HK) surgery on my farsighted patients. Since May 1993, I have presented preliminary findings of my HK procedures to many international ophthalmology meetings. By 1995, I had performed more than 300 HKs. My completed study was published in the March 1995 edition of the *American Journal of Cataract and Refractive Surgery*. I also wrote "Hexagonal Keratotomy," Chapter 17 (pp. 225-231) of <u>Principles and Practice of Refractive Surgery</u> by Richard Elander, published by W. B. Saunders Company in 1997.

The Complete Guide to Refractive Surgery is a comprehensive guide to the correction of refractive errors: nearsightedness, farsightedness, and astigmatism. Also included are chapters on the newest procedures in refractive surgery, including PRK (Excimer Laser), LASIK, and Phakic IOL. The FDA has approved some of these procedures, but not all of them. During the next few years, I will again be at the forefront of ophthalmological advances, when I participate in a core study of Phakic IOLs.

This guide sorts through the information and misinformation to present a focused picture of RK, HK, AK, laser, and implant surgery, American introductions and refinements, criteria for candidacy, the procedures themselves, post-op expectations, care, and complications, lasers in refractive surgery, and the use of computer software to dictate surgery.

Unless otherwise specified, the information that directly relates to case histories, predictability of results, actual results, and success rates relates to my own surgical experience.

Finally, anyone contemplating refractive surgery should make certain that he or she takes care in selecting an ophthalmologist well trained and experienced in performing the needed surgery.

Disclaimer

The author sincerely hopes that *The Complete Guide to Refractive Surgery* will provide useful information for anyone in this country or abroad who is interested in new developments in ophthalmology that could help them or those they love.

Any individual interested in refractive surgery should seek the advice and assistance of a qualified ophthalmologist or ophthalmic surgeon. Before undergoing refractive surgery, the patient should assure himself or herself of the surgeon's appropriate qualifications and experience in the type of refractive surgery chosen. The patient should also make certain that he or she has fully discussed with the surgeon all the alternatives, risks, and complications.

This book provides vital information regarding refractive surgery. The surgical patient's principal source of information, however, should always be his or her chosen ophthalmologist, who can examine the patient and make appropriate medical and surgical determinations.

The author and those who assisted and contributed to the publication of this book cannot be responsible for the medical judgment of physicians who may perform refractive surgery. Neither the author nor his contributors are, nor could they be, responsible for errors in the medical judgment or surgical technique of physicians performing refractive surgery. They cannot be responsible for any complications that may result from the surgery should the reader of this book decide to undergo refractive surgery.

The field of refractive surgery is constantly and rapidly changing, as it is a very young field. The views expressed in this book are my own. Obviously other knowledgeable ophthalmologists may hold different opinions.

Introduction

The use of corrective lenses to improve eyesight spans centuries. In ancient Rome, the use of special magnifying glass balls was, perhaps, the earliest indication of man's attempt to correct vision problems. Subsequent developments throughout Europe set the stage for the eventual creation of eyeglasses and contact lenses.

Ever since, eyeglasses and contact lenses were considered the accepted methods of correcting vision problems.

To discover what charted a new course for ophthalmology worldwide, we must travel to countries far less developed than the United States. Dedicated ophthalmologists in the former USSR and in Mexico have achieved international acclaim for developing microsurgical procedures to correct three of the four most common disorders of refraction: myopia (nearsightedness), hyperopia (farsightedness), and astigmatism. The fourth, presbyopia, is a form of farsightedness caused by aging that is not surgically correctable at this time, although promising research is being done on this problem.

What is refractive surgery, and why the need for *The Complete Guide to Refractive Surgery*?

Refraction, by Webster's definition, is the bending of a ray of light as it passes obliquely from one medium to another. In more simple terms, refraction is the way light focuses from an object through the eye onto the retina. In normal eyes, the focal point is on the retina exactly, responding with a clear image.

In some eyes, however, light rays fall short of the retina (myopia), behind the retina (hyperopia), or are distorted (astigmatism).

Refractive surgery, therefore, involves changing the shape of the cornea to allow light rays to focus on the retina. It can also remove distortion or, most recently, it can involve giving the patient a new lens or using a Phakic IOL, a permanent contact lens.

Most people unfamiliar with the eye care profession are confused about eye problems, who can treat them, and what the treatments are. Myths abound, and misinformation in the media, such as in the early days of RK in the United States, often serves to perpetuate those myths.

To set the record straight about RK and HK, to dispel myths, to offer facts about laser surgery, LASIK, Phakic IOL and Clear Lens Implants, and to clarify other issues in refractive surgery, we decided to re-release *Good-Bye, Glasses* in the expanded edition of *The Complete Guide to Refractive Surgery*. It incorporates all the problems of refraction and the various nonsurgical and surgical corrections. Once again, we have decided to update the earlier edition of *The Complete Guide to Refractive Surgery* with the latest information about refractive surgery procedures.

According to the Opticians Association of America in Fairfax, Virginia, 60 percent of 250 million Americans, as of 1991, needed corrective lenses. The public, particularly that portion that wears corrective lenses for nearsightedness, farsightedness, and/or astigmatism, has the right to know all the options available for correcting their vision problems.

As a specialist in refractive surgery with a long and successful track record, I felt it was my responsibility to help in educating the public so that they can evaluate all options. Herewith, *The Complete Guide to Refractive Surgery, 2nd Edition*.

Stanley C. Grandon, M.D.
Dearborn, Michigan

CHAPTER ONE

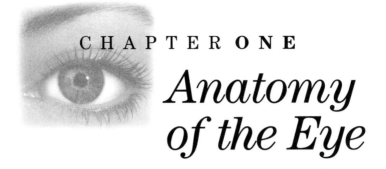

Anatomy of the Eye

The miracle of sight emanates from two small orbs composed of an intricate network of nerves and tiny structures that focus an image on the *retina*. The optic nerves carry a complex flow of impulses stimulated by the retina and crisscross their way to the back section of the brain that controls vision. Both eyes work in conjunction with the brain, which converts the image into electrical impulses. Should the image be less than sharp, the eye can automatically change the focus in a process known as *accommodation*.

The *retina* contains millions of nerve cells that respond to light. The *cornea* and *lens*, focus light, the *pupil* controls the amount of light entering the eye, and the *ciliary body* alters the shape of the lens to adjust the focus. *Fig. 1-a*

The Eyeball

The *orbit*, the bony eye socket that protects the eye from injury, nestles the eyeball in pads of fat. Coordinated by a nerve network in the brain stem, six delicate muscles control each eyeball movement.

The components of the eyeball include: the *sclera*, the tough outer layer more commonly referred to as the white of the

---

[From The American Medical Association's *Home Medical Encyclopedia*, published by Random House, 1989]

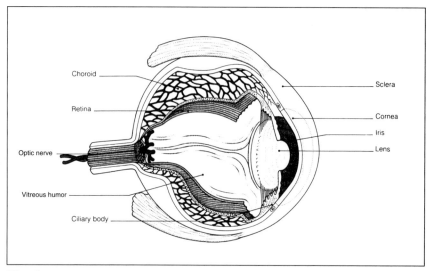

Fig. 1-a

eye; the *cornea*, the slightly protruding clear "window" (the eye's main lens) that performs most of the focusing; the *aqueous humor* (watery fluid) which fills a shallow chamber; the *iris*, behind it, known as the colored part with its *pupil* (central hole), which appears black. In order to control the amount of light entering it, the pupil's size increases or decreases with changes in light intensity.   *Fig. 1-b*

Behind and touching the iris is the *crystalline lens*, suspended by minute fibers from the ciliary body or circular muscle ring. When the ciliary body contracts, the shape of the lens alters to allow focusing power. Vitreous humor, a clear gel, fills the main cavity of the eyeball, behind the lens.

The retina, which rests on the inside of the back of the eye, is a complex composition of nerve tissue that receives images from the cornea and lens. In order to properly function, the retina needs a constant supply of oxygen and sugar. To satisfy this need, a delicate network of blood vessels, *the choroid plexus*, lies immediately under the retina. The *choroid*

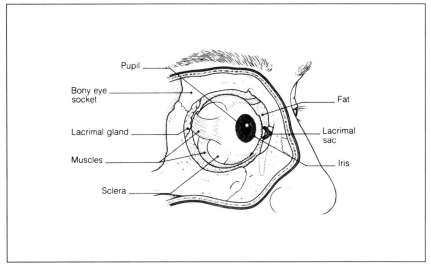

Fig. 1-b

continues at the front of the ciliary body and iris; these three parts make up the *uveal tract*.

The eyeball moves as a result of contraction of one or more of the muscles around it; each of six different muscles pulls the eye in a specific direction.

Conjunctiva

A flexible membrane known as the *conjunctiva* seals off the eyeball from the outside. The conjunctiva is securely attached around the margin of the cornea but rests freely on the sclera over the front third of the eyeball. Attached to the skin at the corners of the eye, the conjunctiva forms the inner lining of the lids, with a deep cul-de-sac above and below. This composition affords a permanent seal while allowing free movement of the eyeball.

The conjunctiva contains many tiny tear-secreting and mucus-producing glands. Along with an oily secretion from the *meibomian glands* in the eyelids, they provide the vital triple layer tear film. That film must constantly cover the cornea and conjunctiva to protect them from damage caused by the drying out of cells.

Eyelids

Each eyelid is home to 30 meibomian glands, their openings running along the lid margin immediately behind the roots of the eyelashes. These glands secrete an oil that prevents lid margin adhesion during sleep and forms the outer layer of the tear film, which prevents evaporation and maintains the continuity of the tear film. The protective reflex of blinking helps to evenly spread the tear film over the cornea. This is crucial for clear vision; a dried-out tear film can cause a corneal abrasion.

Under the skin of the eyelid is a flat, strong muscle that, in an emergency, contracts to push the eyeball back into the orbit and inserts a mass of tissue to protect the eye. This happens as a quick, reflex response to danger.

CHAPTER TWO
The Eye Care Specialists

What is the difference between an optician, an optometrist, and an ophthalmologist? If you do not know, and you face an eye emergency, you could be in for a lot of trouble.

Three kinds of eye care specialists, each with different training and skills, can test eyes and correct vision. They are:

Opticians. Special training enables opticians to fit glasses and contact lenses that an optometrist or an ophthalmologist prescribes.

Optometrists. Trained and licensed to test vision, but not medical doctors, optometrists can prescribe glasses and contact lenses, but usually cannot prescribe medications or treat eye diseases. (This may vary from state to state.) Recently, some states are allowing optometrists to participate in some diagnosis and treatment of eye diseases.

Ophthalmologists. In addition to prescribing glasses, contacts, *and* medications, ophthalmologists, who are medical doctors, specialize in treating eye disorders and performing eye surgery.

In ophthalmology, there are sub-specialties for treating specific parts of the eye and certain eye disorders. Some of the sub-specialists include those who treat retinal problems, diabetes-related disorders, cataracts, glaucoma, and refractive errors. Not all ophthalmologists perform surgery, and surgical skills may vary from ophthalmologist to ophthalmologist.

When should I go to the ophthalmologist?
Even if you are seeing clearly and not experiencing any problems or changes in your vision, you should see an ophthalmologist regularly; at best, once every few years. From the age of 40 and beyond, more frequent examinations are necessary, every other year at least. Some serious eye conditions, such as glaucoma (which can cause blindness), present no symptoms and are diagnosable only by examination. If detected in time, most serious eye conditions can be remedied.

What does an eye examination involve?
Many ophthalmologists employ ophthalmic technicians trained to perform part of the eye examination and assist in surgery. The ophthalmologist looks at each eye through an ophthalmoscope, a slit lamp microscope and other technical instruments that enable him to see the back of the eye for internal eye disorders, such as retinal detachment. With the ophthalmoscope, he can also see if there are any signs of a general disorder, such as anemia, diabetes, or high blood pressure.

If the examiner finds a disorder of refraction, glasses or contacts may be prescribed by the doctor, or surgery may be indicated.

If the doctor and patient concur that surgery is the primary option; then other tests are administered.

The corneal topography and analysis system is a computer-assisted videokeratometer that gives extremely accurate corneal readings and other corneal topography information.

Think of the cornea as a hill, with the corneal topography instrument scanning it from the sky. Some hills have gentle slopes. Other hills have steep inclines on one side and more flat areas on the other side. The corneal topography instrument shows the surgeon the exact locations of the steep and flat parts. It maps out the cornea for astigmatism as well as for LASIK and radial keratotomy.

The instrument has other uses, too. It can aid in fitting contact lenses, because knowing the curvature of the cornea enhances a good fit. Mapping out corneal topography also helps to diagnose early corneal problems, such as keratoconus.

The ultrasound pachymeter, which will be discussed in greater detail in Chapter 6, measures the depth of the cornea. This measurement helps the surgeon determine the depth of the incisions he will make on the surface of the cornea. The ultrasound A-Scan determines the axial length of the eyeball.

Ophthalmic emergencies

Emergencies that involve the eye are not only those that occur when a person is hit in the eye or experiences a foreign object in the eye. Some emergencies know no external origin; for example, a sudden change in or loss of vision, pain in the eye, or flashing lights.

Anyone experiencing these symptoms should see an ophthalmologist immediately or go to the emergency room of a hospital.

CHAPTER THREE

Myopia –
Focusing on the Problem

Most people have good uncorrected vision or need only minor optical corrections to function freely in their everyday lives. For more than 50 percent of the American population, however, corrective lenses — often thick, unattractive ones — are as much a part of their daily wardrobes as clothing and shoes.

If you are nearsighted, you already know what it is like to:

- wake up in the middle of the night and see only a blur of digital lights instead of the distinct readout of your alarm clock;

- swim laps but not be able to time yourself because you cannot read the time on the wall clock — or even see the clock at all;

- work strenuously outdoors in the summer only to have your glasses constantly slide down your sweaty nose; or

- enter a building from the cold, wintry outdoors and not be able to see because your glasses fogged up.

You may have also encountered a life-threatening situation, such as a fire or criminal attack. In the process, you may have been temporarily incapacitated because you broke your glasses or lost your contact lenses and could not see well enough to retrieve them. Or escape imminent danger.

For the person blessed with normal or near-normal vision, identifying with these situations is difficult, if not impossible. Yet they are daily realities for the nearsighted. Reaching for their glasses is one of the first things they do each morning, and removing them is one of the last things they do at night. Between those times, almost everything they do in their occupational and lifestyle situations requires the use of corrective lenses.

Dependence on glasses or contact lenses often limits a person's choice of work, athletic activities, and social pursuits. Many careers are not open to individuals whose uncorrected vision falls below the prescribed level. Military pilots, police officers, fire fighters, and security guards are some of the individuals who must usually meet rigid uncorrected vision requirements.

The nuisance of fogged or slipped glasses or the irritation of contact lenses greatly reduces the enjoyment of athletic activities, such as tennis, jogging, swimming, and skiing.

Many people — particularly those who must wear thick "pop bottle" lenses — suffer lowered self-esteem as a result of their dependence on glasses, and feel socially inhibited.

What is myopia?
Myopia is the medical term for nearsightedness. It means that the eye sees distant objects as blurred or fuzzy. For some people, that distance might be only a foot or two. To help readers with normal vision better understand what the myopic individual sees, look through the lens of a 35mm camera, pretending for a moment that the camera's eye is your own.

Focus a distant object as sharply as possible, indicating how a person with good eyesight sees that object.

Now slowly readjust the focus until the object becomes blurred. The more blurred the object becomes, the more that image parallels the degree of nearsightedness in the myopic person. Seeing that fuzzy image shows you how *everything* appears to the nearsighted whenever he removes his corrective lenses.

What causes myopia?

The cornea, a transparent tissue, serves as a window through which light rays pass on their way to the retina. Myopia results when those light rays fall short of the retina and focus in front of, rather than on, the retina. Often the cornea is so curved that it has too much focusing power. This is myopia. *Fig. 3-a.*

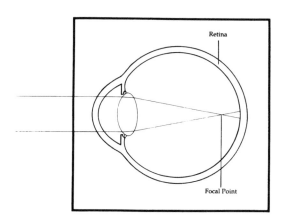

Fig. 3-a   Too much corneal curve causes myopia.

If the curve is lessened or made flat, then light no longer focuses as far forward in the eye, but rather nearer the retina. *Fig. 3-b.*

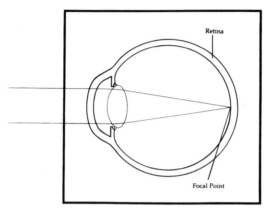

Fig. 3-b   Flattening the corneal curve reduces myopia.

It is generally believed that there is a genetic predisposition to myopia, which may begin any time from early childhood until the late teens. The condition usually stabilizes in the late teens or early 20s.

How is myopia measured?

During a routine examination, an ophthalmologist, optometrist, or ophthalmic technician measures the degree of nearsightedness through a number of specialized tests. A diopter is a measure of myopia.

We commonly refer to vision that is neither nearsighted nor farsighted as 20/20 vision or perfect vision. The larger the bottom [second] number, the more nearsighted the individual is. For example, if a person has -4 diopters of myopia, his vision is more popularly referred to as 20/400. A person is considered legally blind when his vision cannot be corrected with bifocals or contact lenses greater than 20/200. An individual with 20/400 is more myopic than one who is on the borderline of legal blindness.

For the purpose of this book, we define the low range of myopia as -1 to -3 diopters. The middle level extends from -3 (about 20/400) to -6 (20/1200). High myopes fall above -6. High degrees of myopia are so difficult to measure that the examiner must resort to a simple "show and tell" test. In that test, the patient counts the number of fingers the examiner holds up at different distances. We refer to this method as the "count fingers" test.

CHAPTER FOUR
Hyperopia and Astigmatism

Myopia and hyperopia are refractive conditions with opposite effects. Individuals with myopia see near objects clearly; those with hyperopia see distant objects clearly.

If you are farsighted, you know what it is like to:

- reach for your glasses before you can read the morning paper, a good novel, or a restaurant menu;

- need your glasses to be able to see where to sign an application for a job, a loan, or a credit card;

- put your glasses on before you can thread a needle or do most handiwork or crafts; or

- require glasses to be able to work at your computer at home or on the job.

For the farsighted, the pleasures of reading, working a crossword puzzle, knitting, or baiting a hook diminish every time they forget or misplace their glasses.

What is hyperopia?

Hyperopia, or farsightedness, is a condition that causes a point in space to focus behind the retina.

Often, farsighted individuals can see distant objects clearly but have difficulty reading. As a hyperopic person ages, he can also lose distance vision, because the eye loses its ability to change as easily.

When you are young, your eye can accommodate the shape of its lens easier, making the eye stronger. However, the more you age, the more the lens stiffens, and therefore the more it loses its ability to change shape.

People who have been glasses-free all their lives greatly dislike depending on them when farsightedness occurs. When they are that uncomfortable, they will do almost anything to eliminate their need for glasses.

What is the difference between hyperopia and presbyopia?

Often, when a person is farsighted, he needs corrective lenses for both distance and near vision. When one is presbyopic, however, only the near vision needs correction.

There is physiologically increasing difficulty in older people to visually accommodate (naturally focus on near and far objects). The medical term for this problem is *presbyopia*. It is the reason why there are so many bifocal prescriptions for people over the age of 40.

With the development of hexagonal keratotomy (HK), farsighted people were able to utilize any of the options available for myopic people: eyeglasses, contact lenses, and surgery.

Presbyopic individuals, on the other hand, cannot find relief from their farsighted condition through surgery. If we could do that, we would find the cure for aging. [Note: Miracle of miracles! An ophthalmologist in Texas by the name of Ronald

A. Schachar, M.D., is working on developing a surgical procedure to correct presbyopia. Although the procedure may not be ready for the public for many years, it does show possible promise.]

What causes hyperopia?

When the eye is too short from front to back, or when there is a weakness in the focusing power of the lens or cornea [the clear "window" at the front of the eye] the result is hyperopia. The focal point of parallel lights in a farsighted person is behind the retina. *Fig. 4-a.* Hyperopia generally is present from birth and usually is diagnosed in early childhood. Hyperopia tends to run in families, and it gets worse with age.

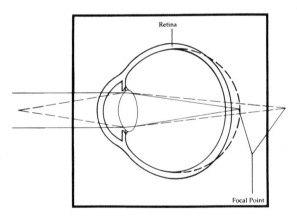

Fig. 4-a The farsighted (hyperopic) eye focuses images behind the retina.

What are the symptoms of hyperopia?

Many people with mild farsightedness have no symptoms. Others experience eye strain (an aching in the eye) due to constant use of certain eye muscles to focus more clearly. People with moderate to severe hyperopia have continuously blurred vision and may also have eye strain. Neither symptom damages the vision permanently.

How is hyperopia treated in early stages?
If farsightedness is not severe, a young eye can accommodate the condition and overcome it naturally. This occurs by the lens changing shape and increasing its focusing power. As the person gets older, the lens does not change shape easily, and he needs glasses for distance and near vision.

How is hyperopia treated in later stages?
If eye examinations conducted by an ophthalmologist indicate you are farsighted, you may elect to wear eyeglasses or contact lenses, or you might have qualified for hexagonal keratotomy (HK), a surgical procedure that corrected farsightedness. Hexagonal keratotomy was a very good operation. However, some refractive surgeons, not trained in the proper techniques, performed a form of the operation that resulted in complications. As a result, very few surgeons are now performing hexagonal keratotomy. Phakic IOL, a new procedure that shows promise for correcting hyperopia, is discussed in Chapter 17. Another new procedure, involving clear lens implants, is being done in Florida. In it, the surgeon takes out the human lens and implants a more powerful folding lens that allows an image to focus on the retina. The procedure is discussed in Chapter 18. Now, LASIK is being done for hyperopia. The results are early, but they show promise. LASIK surgery for the correction of hyperopia will be discussed in Chapter 16.

What is astigmatism?
Astigmatism, or distorted vision, is a condition in which vertical lines might be in focus, but not horizontal lines, or vice versa. Diagonal lines might also be out of focus. Distant points in space become a blur on the retina. *Fig. 4-b.*

CHAPTER FOUR   HYPEROPIA AND ASTIGMATISM | 19

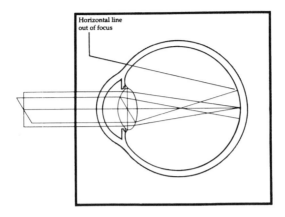

Fig. 4-b A cornea that is not spherical causes astigmatism.

A person can have a little or a lot of astigmatism. Sometimes it occurs in conjunction with nearsightedness or farsightedness. Astigmatism usually is present from birth, and it may change with age.

What causes astigmatism?
Uneven curvature of the cornea causes astigmatism. It results when one axis is stronger than the other, causing a blurring on the retina. In other words, one axis focuses differently than the other. High astigmatism can cause double or ghost images.

How do we measure astigmatism?
A keratometer determines the degree of astigmatism by measuring each of the curves of the cornea separately. A measure of astigmatism is also known as a diopter.

What is the treatment for astigmatism?
If an eye examination reveals astigmatism, glasses or hard contact lenses, shaped to the curvature needed to correct the unevenness of the cornea, may be prescribed. These will enable the person to see normally.

Can surgery correct astigmatism?
Astigmatic keratotomy (a variation of the surgery that corrects myopia and hyperopia) can be performed to correct astigmatism by itself. However, if a person is considering having surgery to correct nearsightedness, his or her surgeon may be able to perform additional surgery at the same time to correct astigmatism. LASIK can also be used to correct astigmatism.

CHAPTER FIVE
Non-Surgical Treatments

There are three recognized non-surgical treatments of refractive conditions:

- eyeglasses

- contact lenses

- and an additional non-surgical treatment of myopia: orthokeratology.

Eyeglasses

Eyeglasses, or spectacles as they were once known, have been and still are the most common method of correcting myopic, hyperopic, and astigmatic vision. For the most part, they are safe, but some people dislike their appearance in glasses, find they interfere with their work, or are bothered by wearing them in athletic activities or social situations. In cases of high myopia, glasses needed for sufficient correction may be thick and have the tendency to minimize image size by as much as 25 percent, in some cases.

The primary benefit of eyeglasses is the relatively inexpensive way of obtaining a certain amount of correction. The availability of different styles of lenses and frames allows the individual to coordinate glasses with the entire wardrobe.

For all the benefits glasses give, they also present some drawbacks:

- Glasses cannot give completely *normal* vision. If you look at any object through a piece of glass — even a window — you will notice that there can be some distortion and color change.

- Eyeglasses represent a certain annoyance to the eyes. Most people have to adjust to wearing glasses, particularly bifocals, and patients with high myopia have great difficulty becoming accustomed to a full-correction.

- Strong lenses required for correcting high myopia minify the objects a person sees. They make them appear smaller than they really are.

- Glasses can limit the field of vision to the size of the lens. Even patients with weak glasses cannot see clearly unless they look through the center of the lenses.

- Keeping glasses clean is one of the minor but ever-present annoyances associated with this form of correction. Damp, rainy conditions fog the lenses. Hot weather causes them to have a similar effect. Cold temperatures cause glasses to become cloudy by the moisture of one's breath or when one enters a warm place. And dust and smudges rarely make glasses the clear windows they are supposed to be.

- Likewise, reflections of strong light from eyeglasses are often annoying. Some patients complain that one-on-one eye contact is virtually impossible whenever glare "whites out" the eyes of the person wearing glasses.

- Some people consider eyeglasses to be disfiguring, a matter of minor consideration perhaps in light of the benefit they offer. Psychological comfort and a healthy self-image, however, are vital to the overall well-being of an individual.

- Since myopia changes over a person's lifetime (usually substantially stabilizing by about age 18), eyeglass prescriptions must be regularly checked and updated. Those changes require the purchase of new prescription lenses, not to mention keeping up with the latest fashions in frames.

The contact lens alternative

Hard and soft contact lenses are becoming a more and more popular alternative to eyeglasses for the correction of refractive errors. In certain instances, contacts offer major optical advantages over glasses. Contacts, however, are not tolerated by some people.

Many companies worldwide make various types of contact lenses. The lens was declared a medical device and is therefore controlled by the Food & Drug Administration in the United States. Some contact lenses have a very high water content (as much as 70 percent) and can be worn for as long as one week at a time. However, some soft contact lenses do not completely correct high degrees of astigmatism. There are now special designs available to correct most degrees of astigmatism.

Gas permeable lenses

Other plastic materials have been used which have increased gas permeability. Silicone lenses have superior oxygen and carbon dioxide permeability.

Gas permeable lenses are a compromise between the original hard contact lenses and soft lenses. Permitting oxygen and carbon dioxide to pass through them to and from the eyes, gas permeable lenses offer the sharp vision of hard lenses but with better oxygen transport. They usually suit individuals who cannot tolerate standard hard lenses, but who are unable to use soft lenses because of certain vision problems.

Bifocal contact lenses
Bifocal contact lenses are primarily for people 40 or older who need a lens for close-up reading as well as one for distance.

Bifocal soft contacts have a zone in the center of the lens for distance viewing and an outer or bottom one for reading. They come in hard, soft, and gas permeable materials. Like bifocal glasses, these lenses take some adjusting to, and they will not satisfy every bifocal wearer's needs.

Tinted contact lenses
Soft and gas permeable tinted contacts were approved by the FDA for people who want to change or enhance the natural color of their eyes. (Tinted hard contacts have been available for more than 30 years.) Deeper tints have clear centers for normal light transmission.

Extended wear contacts and corneal ulcers
Short-term, extended wear contact lenses are now available, but many cases of corneal ulcers — some causing complete loss of vision — have been reported.

In the November 8, 1985, edition of *The Wall Street Journal*, a report stated that some ophthalmologists were concerned about the safety of extended wear contact lenses. At that time, the FDA had approved the use of extended wear contacts for up to 30 days without removal, even during sleep.

About five million Americans now wear the lenses, and for a while their sales grew faster than any other type of corrective lenses.

According to the article, however, there was concern that these extended wear contact lenses were not as safe as they were once thought to be. The trouble was that an increasing, but still very small, number of corneal ulcers was being detected in extended wear contact lens users. A corneal ulcer occurs when the surface of the cornea (known as the *epithelium*) is deprived of oxygen, is scraped or scarred, and bacteria and pus pockets form. In rare, severe cases, infection punctures the epithelium, usually resulting in partial or full loss of vision, depending on the location of the ulcer in the cornea.

The article also reports that Louis Wilson, a professor of ophthalmology at Emory University School of Medicine and one of the foremost experts on extended wear contact lenses, cautions that the full extent of the problem has yet to be determined. He and other experts say thousands of corneal ulcer cases were reported among users of extended wear contact lenses since 1981, when the FDA approved them for cosmetic, rather than strictly therapeutic, use. Of those thousands of cases, they report, probably 100 or less have been so severe that the cornea was destroyed or that the individual became legally blind.

FDA warning

In 1989, the FDA asked makers of extended wear contact lenses and disposable lenses to relabel them for continuous use of no longer than seven days. The agency said current labeling — allowing for up to 30 days of continuous wear — presented too high a risk of developing a potentially vision-damaging disease called *ulcerative keratitis* (infection of the cornea that can be painful and destroy vision). That risk is about six times greater for extended wear lens users than for people with daily wear lenses.

Data from a study sponsored by the Contact Lens Institute "did not identify a wearing time that will eliminate the risk altogether," said FDA Commissioner Frank E. Young, M.D., Ph.D. "However, seven days represents a relatively short, easy-to-remember interval, which will encourage users to remove their lenses and clean them."

Care and use of contact lenses

When it has been determined that a person can safely wear extended wear contact lenses, proper instruction in the care, insertion, removal, and cleaning is imperative to avoid any complications. If the eye becomes red, the person should remove the lens immediately. Irritations or a change in vision represents other signs of trouble that contact lens wearers often ignore.

Although the FDA has approved the use of extended wear contact lenses for up to seven days without removal, many ophthalmologists recommend daily cleaning.

Handling a contact lens is difficult for some people. Wearers must daily insert and remove lenses and change them throughout the day to wash away dust particles than can irritate the eyes. Compliance in the care of all types of contact lenses is important. Poor maintenance is usually the cause of most contact lens related problems.

Orthokeratology

The third non-surgical treatment of myopia is a technique that involves wearing a successive series of hard contact lenses that mechanically flatten the curvature of the cornea. This technique mandates the use of so-called "retainer" lenses at regular intervals to maintain this flatness so that the patient can see without the lenses for varying periods of time. Not all patients are eligible for orthokeratology for many reasons, and some people have experienced intolerance prior to the fitting of the retainer lenses.

Orthokeratology is generally useful only in cases of very mild myopia.

Surgical alternatives to RK

Although this chapter presents the non-surgical treatments of refractive conditions, four relatively new surgical procedures also bear mention:

Keratomileusis

During this procedure, a very thin layer of the cornea is removed, lathe-cut, and sutured back onto the cornea. While there may be some advantages for extremely high myopes, there may be greater risk potential with this operation than with other procedures, and fewer cases have been performed.

Automated Lamellar Keratoplasty (ALK)

In the ALK procedure for hyperopia, the surgeon cuts through 70 percent of the corneal depth to create a corneal bulge that causes corneal steepening and affects correction of the farsightedness.

For myopia, the surgeon makes a non-refractive incision through 30 percent of the corneal depth. He then makes another incision, the refractive cut, behind the front one, creating a flap. He then places the cornea back on, and also replaces the flap. Compared to RK, this procedure carries increased risk.

Epikeratophakia

This surgical procedure, which holds some advantages for high myopes, involves making a groove in the cornea and suturing a donor corneal tissue that has been lathe-cut. There have been some problems with accuracy with this procedure, particularly in patients losing best corrected vision.

Lasers

In photorefractive keratoplasty, or PRK as it is more commonly known, a "cold" laser carves the cornea into a new shape. The problem with this procedure is that the laser severs a membrane (known as Bowman's membrane) in the front of the eye. No one knows the long-term effect of the eye without Bowman's membrane, as this procedure was never done before. In keratomileusis, ALK, and LASIK, Bowman's membrane is displaced but later put back. In laser surgery, the membrane is gone forever and its removal can even cause permanent decreased visual acuity. If you cut too deeply into the *stroma* (the middle of the cornea), corneal haze or scarring results. These problems can cause such visual symptoms as glare and distortion, and can even cause decreased visual acuity.

The Food & Drug Administration has approved the Excimer Laser (PRK) procedure for use in the United States for up to -12 diopters of myopia and three to four diopters of astigmatism. With PRK there is a surface ablation as up to one-third of the cornea is removed by a laser. The procedure is quite painful, and postoperative complications include light sensitivity, glare, irregular astigmatism, and hazing.

With LASIK, there is very little pain, faster healing time, and fewer postoperative complications with glare and hazing. Some problems with corneal flaps have occurred, which is one of the disadvantages of this procedure. However, with the newer Keratome technology (flapmaker), flap problems are seldom seen.

The beauty of radial keratotomy is that the surgeon does not touch the *visual axis* (the center of the cornea through which you see). As a result, it is rare that there is any substantial loss of visual acuity. With the surface laser and ALK procedures, the surgeon cuts through the visual axis, so any healing irregularities or hazing causes irregular astigmatism that cannot be corrected with glasses. Any scarring causes loss of best corrected visual acuity. With LASIK's improving technology, again, loss of best corrected visual acuity is becoming a rare occurrence.

The subject of lasers in refractive surgery will be discussed in greater detail in Chapters 14, 15, and 16 of this book.

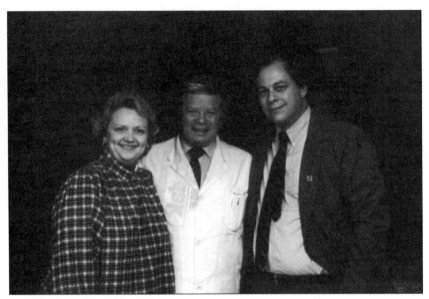
Authors Susan Giffin, left and Dr. Stanley C. Grandon, right, with Professor Svyatoslav Fyodorov in Moscow, 1986.

CHAPTER SIX

RK –
A Surgical Solution, Soviet-Style

Radial keratotomy is not cosmetic surgery. You can be a pilot if you have a badly shaped nose, but you cannot be a pilot if your eyesight is poor.

– S. Fyodorov

The gray marble building, headquarters for the Moscow Research Institute of Eye Microsurgery, projected a monochromatic tableau against a cloudy Moscow morning sky. Inside, the theme continued: gray marble floors, gray marble walls…everywhere. A small elevator, typical of those in Moscow hotels and office buildings, carried us up to Professor Svyatoslav Fyodorov's office suite. A friendly Soviet doctor, who spoke good English, greeted us and showed us to the conference room. She shared some of the literature produced by the institute, where they developed modern radial keratotomy.

With the aid of a highly proficient interpreter, we proceeded to tour one floor after another before we met Fyodorov, known as the father of radial keratotomy.

Each floor was a bustle of activity. Patients, often dressed in the poor street clothes of country folk, lined the corridors awaiting their turn for eye examinations, treatments of various eye disorders, or surgery. Smiles that bared gold or silver teeth flashed every now and then as the American guests passed by.

It was here in this environment...not in the slick, high tech laboratories of the western world...that radial keratotomy was developed. Ironically, the seeds were planted in 1970 in, of all places, a movie theater on Broadway in New York City! Fyodorov told his own story:

It was my first trip to the United States. I was in New York City and was dazzled by all the bright lights of Broadway, so I decided to see a movie there. The film was Woody Allen's "Sleeper," in which all of the action takes place in the year 2100. Everything is different — clothes, homes, sex, transportation, everything, except glasses. At the time, I thought, 'If everything else can change by the year 2100, why can't the need for glasses change?'

Not long after Fyodorov returned to Moscow, he found an opportunity to answer that question. "A doctor at our Moscow clinic brought to me a boy of 18, who had been injured in a school yard scuffle," recalled Fyodorov. "The nearsighted young man wore glasses and, in the course of fighting, his glasses broke, and a piece of the lens lacerated one of his corneas. A few days later, he came to me and said, 'Dr. Fyodorov! I can see with my eye without wearing my glasses!'

Fyodorov then realized that if an accidental cut on the cornea could correct myopia, he could devise a surgical procedure to accomplish the same result deliberately. He instructed his young surgeons to begin experimental surgery on the corneas of rabbits. "We worked for one and a half years with rabbits," said Fyodorov. "After three to five months, we found every rabbit cornea had become more flat by two to three diopters after 10 to 16 incisions. We learned that when we made more than 16 incisions, we got no greater results, so we decided to make a maximum of 16 incisions."

CHAPTER SIX — RK – A SURGICAL SOLUTION, SOVIET-STYLE

In 1973, Misha Tytsuna, a young driver for the clinic, became the first human to undergo Fyodorov's radial keratotomy procedure. "Misha had -3 diopters of myopia," said Fyodorov. He performed the operation of 16 incisions freehand with a small piece of a razor blade. "I was a little nervous." The operation was a success, and today, 25 years later, Misha has 20/25 vision in both eyes.

When confident he was on the right track, Fyodorov continued performing radial keratotomies. To control the amount of flattening of the cornea, he made the optical zone smaller. (The optical zone or visual axis is the central part of the cornea through which you see. By making radial incisions on the surface of the cornea, the optical zone — or clear zone — is flattened, enabling light to focus nearer the retina than it did before surgery.)

By 1974, Fyodorov had performed successfully 104 radial keratotomy operations. "All the patients had had -2 to -4 diopters of myopia," he said, "and all achieved excellent results."

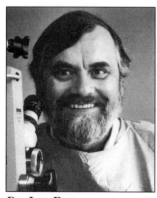
Dr. Leo Bores

From 1975 to 1976, Fyodorov performed more than 700 cases, all with very good results, according to Fyodorov. During that time, Dr. Leo Bores, an ophthalmologist from Wayne State University in Detroit, Michigan, visited Moscow to observe Fyodorov's technique for intraocular lens implants for cataract surgery. "When Fyodorov and I met, it was as if we'd known each other for a hundred years," said Bores. "It was one of those instant things. He showed me his intraocular lens technique. He also showed me his radial keratotomy procedure, known then as the *dosage dissection of the circumferential ligament of Cucote*. I was intrigued. While I was in Moscow, I performed this operation on 12 or 13 patients. In 1977, when I returned to Moscow, I checked the results of those patients. I was very satisfied, so in November, 1978, I did the first case in the United States."

His first radial keratotomy patient was a pleasant young woman named Gwen, who worked for American Airlines. "She originally came to me because she couldn't wear glasses comfortably," Bores said. "We tried to fit her with contact lenses, but it seemed all we ever got was grief.

"When I returned from my first trip to Moscow I 1976, I saw Gwen on a routine visit to my office about yet another contact lens problem. I said, 'Gwen, if you don't knock off this stuff, I'm going to have to cut your eyes like the Russians do.' She kept bugging me and bugging me. So, in 1978, I did her."

Bores performed surgery on Gwen's eyes about two weeks apart. "She turned out fantastic," he said. "I didn't know until she was interviewed on *CBS Morning News* exactly how much effect it had had on her life, although I had an inkling. After surgery on her second eye, she came to my office. My secretary came back to me and said, 'Dr. Bores, Gwen is outside, but you must see her to believe it.' She was a totally new person. Totally. Her hair was different. The way she stood was different. The way she talked was different. The way she dressed was different. She said, 'I'm free!' I kidded her, and she said, 'Yeah, I know how they felt. I could sing and be real spiritual, because that's how I feel now…free!'"

Although the first operation performed in the United States was successful, Bores was in for some rough sledding as the procedure gained recognition. In April 1979, Fyodorov visited the United States and held a press conference in Washington, D.C., on myopia surgery. *"The Detroit Free Press* interviewed me after that news broke, and that's when everything hit the fan," Bores recalled.

The problem revolved around the fact that due to the nature of the American medical system, new procedures have a difficult time gaining acceptance by the medical profession. Most of the new procedures come from outside the United States.

"Ironically, the situation in American medicine is a disease process," explained Bores. "Defective thinking. A famous surgeon says there is a process which surgeons go through. First of all, surgeons are very conservative. When they first see something that's new, they'll say it's not good. Then when they find out it's good, they'll say it's not true. When they find out it's true, they'll say it's not new. And when they've assimilated all that, they convince themselves that they started it."

After Bores performed the first radial keratotomy in the United States, he thought American ophthalmologists would rally 'round him because they would feel so good about this revolutionary procedure. "Wrong!" said Bores. "I thought I was going to be barbecued over green twigs. And then I realized what was happening. I said to myself, 'You are a student of history, but you're not paying attention to it. What happened to Morgan when he brought chloroform anesthesia back to the United States? They wanted to lynch him; he barely escaped with his life. Louis Pasteur, the same. Anybody who has had a new idea in medicine has been treated like dirt."

That is what happened to Bores. "A lot of people have convinced themselves that they were on the ground floor of radial keratotomy in this country but they weren't. As a matter of fact, almost everyone backed away, because no one wanted to be around when the bombs started to fall," he said. "You know, close counts only in horseshoes and hand grenades. Very few people wanted to stand close to me.

"The problem is that we used to be very innovative people in America. We used to be pioneering and very aggressive, but no one wants to take responsibility for anything we do. Any time a doctor does something and it doesn't work — remember, doctors are supposed to be miracle workers — he gets his pants sued off. Well, that's enough to scare anyone. You know, twice burned, twice wise.

"American medicine is going the way European medicine went," Bores continued. "You're going to see stagnation. Everything is going to die. All the energy will croak, and there will be no new things.

"The fact that radial keratotomy came from the Soviet Union is an absolute miracle. They have a dead medical culture there. Anything new in the future might come out of Fyodorov's clinic. Maybe. But not out of the rest of the Soviet Union."

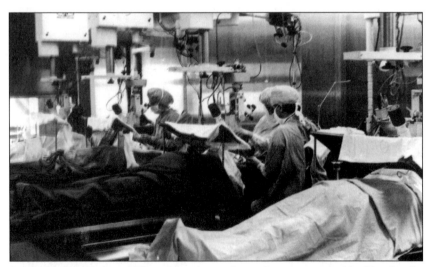

In the Soviet Union, RK surgery is performed on an assembly-line basis.

CHAPTER SEVEN
RK – *American Refinements*

America's pioneering days in medicine may have passed, but when it comes to improving and refining techniques developed abroad, American ingenuity is still alive and well.

The name of the Soviet procedure was one of the first changes made by American ophthalmologists. Bores and Dr. William D. Myers, a Detroit ophthalmologist who worked with Bores in the early days of radial keratotomy in the United States, decided Fyodorov's name for the procedure was too cumbersome. "We thought that since we were cutting the cornea with radial incisions, we should call the procedure *radial keratotomy* or RK for short," explained Bores. "We introduced that term in May, 1980, at a meeting at the Kresge Eye Institute in Detroit. Fyodorov loved it."

That same year, Dr. Leeds Katzen, the third ophthalmologist to perform radial keratotomy in the United States, helped organize the first course in RK surgery, in Baltimore, Maryland.

When radial keratotomy was introduced in the United States, as it was performed in the Soviet Union, surgeons did not have the advantages of ultrasound pachymetry, the diamond knife or computer predictability software, the three greatest — and largely American — contributions to RK surgery. In those days, surgeons measured corneal thickness with an optic pachymeter, and did the cutting with a metal blade.

The cornea is like a sponge. It absorbs water very quickly. Like fine French pastry. One of the early modifications in the Soviet RK procedures was that Bores did not wet the cornea. [Actually, Myers originated the idea of performing RK on a dry cornea.] "The results changed when we didn't wet the cornea," Bores said. "The cornea cut differently. It didn't swell up."

In both the United States and the Soviet Union, the search was underway for improvements, and sometimes they were discovered almost simultaneously.

Measuring the cornea with ultrasound

At an ophthalmology meeting in 1980, Bores met a young ophthalmologist by the name of Dr. Fred Kremer, Philadelphia, Pennsylvania, who mentioned it might be possible to measure the cornea with ultrasound. From that notion eventually came the D.G.H. 2000, which is programmable and which is, according to Bores, the state-of-the-art in ultrasound pachymetry today. It has been one of the greatest contributions to RK surgery, because it allows the surgeon to more accurately measure corneal thickness and to subsequently map the incisions he will make during surgery.

Cutting with diamonds

At the same meeting, another important break in American RK surgery came when Dr. Dennis Shepard, Santa Maria, California, demonstrated the advantages of the blue blade over a stainless steel blade. "It was sharper. It cut deeper, and we began to get corrections in patients as high as eight diopters," Bores explained.

RK surgeons were still not convinced that they had found the best instrument for making the delicate radial incisions. In 1981, Fyodorov discovered that a diamond could serve as the best "knife" for RK surgery. "It's not easy making a diamond for surgery," Fyodorov explained, "because it is difficult to polish a diamond to the desired sharpness. But the people of Urkutia, USSR, where diamonds are mined, discovered it is possible to polish diamonds with a combination of temperature and a special chemistry. With this treatment, the diamond melts like ice and can be made very sharp, something that cannot be accomplished with any polishing machine, because the vibrations can easily destroy the diamond by chipping. That's why we made the diamond knife, and the results of our surgeries improved immediately."

The diamond knife with micrometer handle

In the United States, at about the same time, according to Bores, KOI, a small manufacturer of contact lenses, developed the first American diamond knife. "It was based on the trifacet blade," said Bores. "I used it, but found that over time the diamond knife was inconsistent, so I went back to steel blades that had been cut with a laser and honed. We tried many other materials to make better blades — obsidian, ceramic, and ruby, which was terrible. Finally, the very sharpest blades I found were made of sapphire, but they could not be easily manufactured because they were too fragile. And the sapphire blade was expensive — $400. It was good for at least 10 cases, maybe more. It became very popular, but not many people use it today, because they are enamored of the diamond."

Bores still prefers the sapphire blade, but the present state-of-the-art diamond knife with the micrometer handle that allows the surgeon to set the depth of the blade has prevailed.

Predicting RK results

As far back as 1979, Fyodorov began using a computer for calculations in RK surgery. Due, in part, to the large volume of RK surgery performed in the United States over what was being done in the Soviet Union, American ophthalmologists advanced the use of computers in documenting RK results. Today, highly sophisticated computer software aids refractive surgeons.

Establishing credibility

According to Bores, by 1981, there still were no quality data in medical literature from groups investigating radial keratotomy. To obtain this needed information for the Analytical Radial Keratotomy Study Group (also known as the ARK Study Group), several ophthalmic surgeons in private practice devised data-collection systems in their offices. These systems gathered perspective data on all of their RK patients. All of the surgeons in this group used well-defined surgical protocols.

After performing the procedure, the surgeons involved in the ARK Study Group filed reports showing the number of incisions made, estimated depth, and size of the clear zone. Surgeons conducted as many as eight follow-up examinations in the first postoperative year of the study.

According to Dr. Donald R. Sanders, associate professor of ophthalmology at the University of Illinois Eye and Ear Infirmary at Chicago, more than 500 cases reached the one-year follow-up mark in the ARK Study. No surgically related complications, which resulted in a significant loss of best corrected visual acuity, were reported. Postoperative, uncorrected visual acuity was 20/40 or better in 74 percent of the cases. Among patients who had less than -6 diopters of myopia postoperatively, vision improved to 20/40 or better in 83 percent. Thirty-five percent achieved 20/20 or better vision.

By 1983, the ARK Study Group had been in existence for two years. The National Institute of Health had partly funded the study federally, beginning in February 1982. Three centers around the country collected the data; and by May 1983, clinics had amassed data on more than 2,000 RK cases. Sanders, a renowned ophthalmic researcher in the United States, and Ronald G. Marks, Ph.D., associate professor of biostatistics at the University of Florida, Gainesville, provided scientific corroboration and support.

Surgeons who participated in the ARK Study Group were Dr. Harold Sawelson, Florida; Dr. Peter Arrowsmith, Tennessee; and Dr. Michael Dietz, Pennsylvania. They gained considerable respect for the importance of data collection under a specific protocol. (I became an adjunct investigator for the ARK Study Group in 1982, shortly before it disbanded.)

"When the information starts pouring out, the credibility attached to that data can make a whole different approach to your thinking," said Bores, "and you know you're receiving good information. The ARK Study Group approach was very solid, and it led to more understanding of the RK procedure and its predictability much faster than other types of studies that weren't closely monitored by such people."

In 1982, the ARK Study Group reported valuable clinical data on the procedure. This data seriously impacted the analysis and evaluation of RK surgery and, along with other developments in the procedure, influenced the acceptance of radial keratotomy in the United States.

Changing the status of RK surgery

The American Academy of Ophthalmology in July 1980, stated that radial keratotomy was "experimental and should be the subject of additional, carefully controlled studies before widespread adoption." In the fall of 1983, the Academy stated that RK was an "investigational" procedure.

The National Eye Institute funded a five-year, nationwide Prospective Evaluation of Radial Keratotomy (the PERK Study). In late 1984, the PERK Study released its results, which confirmed what other studies, including the ARK Study, had already shown. The PERK Study results were quite good, although the ARK Study results were even better.

Through the years of improvements, refinements, data collections, and analyses, radial keratotomy in the United States has evolved as an accepted alternative for the treatment of myopia.

In 1986, Dr. George O. Waring III, who directed the PERK Study, made these conclusions:

The results of the radial keratotomy studies that have been undertaken since 1980 — including the ARK Study and the PERK Study — show that, under appropriate circumstances and for qualified patients, radial keratotomy is effective in reducing myopia. Enough data is now available to establish that radial keratotomy is not an 'experimental' procedure. It is a new addition to the list of alternatives available to treat myopia.

Further, in 1988, Waring released the following statement:

A few hundred thousand radial keratotomy procedures have been performed by approximately 10 percent of American ophthalmologists. A wealth of clinical and laboratory data has now defined a relative level of safety and effectiveness for the procedure.

The PERK Study released its final results in the February 23, 1990, issue of the *Journal of the American Medical Association (JAMA)*. According to the report, 76 percent of those who had radial keratotomy on both eyes had a result of 20/40 uncorrected vision or better.

"A major drawback of radial keratotomy surgery is the inability of the surgeon to accurately predict the outcome for an individual eye," the researchers noted.

With the development of sophisticated computer software, some radial keratotomy surgeons now are able to predict the outcome of surgery with quite good accuracy. See Chapter 19 for more information on computers in RK surgery.

In the final analysis, the study found, radial keratotomy, which improved vision in most recipients, is now considered relatively safe and more effective than it was when introduced in the United States 15 years earlier.

In 1995, the PERK Study came out with further findings. In general, the results were similar to those in 1990, but in some cases there was a very small amount of hyperopic shifting over many years. Some other studies agreed with this; still others did not.

The status of RK surgery in 1999

RK surgery, which has now been performed successfully on more than one million eyes in the United States alone, is an almost completely safe procedure. In fact, it is one of the safest procedures in medicine today. The complication rate remains extremely low; in my own 16,000 cases, very few people have ever lost even one or two best corrected lines of vision. As of this writing in 1999, I rarely perform radial keratotomy on patients with -6 or more diopters of myopia. For patients with up to -6 diopters of myopia, radial keratotomy works well. Lately, I have been encouraging patients from -4 to -6 diopters to also consider LASIK (or, for that matter, any lower myope who wants it).

As LASIK becomes more technologically advanced, more people will probably opt for LASIK, as it has some advantages over radial keratotomy (such as almost no pain, immediate restoration of improved vision, increased accuracy, and no fluctuation of vision). Suffice it to say, on the other hand, that radial keratotomy is an almost totally safe procedure. The safety record in the experienced surgeon's hands is unequaled. For individuals with -3 and lower degrees of myopia, approximately 99% achieve 20/40 or better with RK surgery in good hands.

With Fyodorov, refractive surgery was an infant. Now, as Bores likes to say, the baby is an adolescent. For any procedure to become accepted, one generation must pass. We celebrate, in 1999, radial keratotomy's silver anniversary, 25 years or more than a generation, since Fyodorov performed the first RK on human eyes, those of his driver, Misha. So the controversy has ended, at long last.

One of the best side effects of RK surgery has been that the procedure has led to many other advances in ophthalmology worldwide. Surgeons from all over the world are contributing to the advancement of ophthalmology.

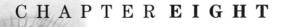

CHAPTER EIGHT
HK and AK –
Mexican Developments, American Refinements

[As a matter of historical reference, we are including the relatively short history of hexagonal keratotomy. This procedure is rarely, if ever, being performed any longer in the United States.]

Just as radial keratotomy was developed outside the United States, so were the procedures that correct farsightedness and astigmatism.

So, too, did American ophthalmologists refine all three procedures — radial keratotomy, hexagonal keratotomy, and astigmatic keratotomy.

You have just read the fascinating story of the Soviet development of radial keratotomy and the magnificent vision Dr. Bores had to bring this revolutionary procedure to the United States.

Fortunately, for the later development of HK and AK surgery, the battles waged for acceptance of RK surgery have made it immensely easier for HK and AK to become accepted by the American ophthalmologic community. A significant part of that ease of acceptance was the similarity of the procedures. Basically, the principal difference is the variation of the surgical pattern.

Hexagonal keratotomy

The microsurgical procedure that corrects farsightedness originated with Dr. Antonio Mendez of Mexico in 1985. His procedure consisted of making a connected hexagonal design on the surface of the cornea. With this procedure there were some healing problems with the incisions. *Fig. 8-a.*

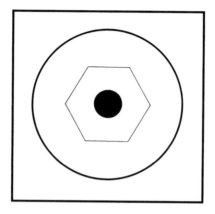

Fig. 8-a   Mendez's connected hexagon for the correction of hyperopia

American surgeons later realized that they could achieve the same result and make the eye stronger if they disconnected the hexagon. However, the amount of results decreased. *Fig. 8-b.*

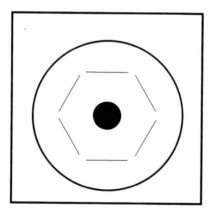

Fig. 8-b   American disconnected hexagon

As one of the first American ophthalmologists to perform a long series of hexagonal keratotomy (HK) procedures, I entered into a formal study with Sanders, a brilliant statistician. Participating with Sanders in a study bodes well for the acceptance of the statistics and research methodology, but does not influence the acceptance of the surgical procedure itself or the results of surgery.

In my own experience, I used the surgical pattern of not only Mendez but also of other American ophthalmologists. My surgical pattern for hexagonal keratotomy consisted of six incisions in a disconnected spiral hexagon, leaving a five- to six-millimeter optical zone, as opposed to a three-millimeter optical zone for radial keratotomy. *Fig. 8-c.*

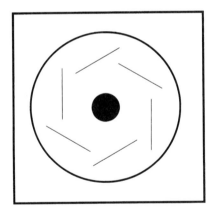

Fig. 8-c   Grandon's disconnected spiral hexagon

The gaps between incisions had to be equal, and the amount of space after each incision also had to be equal. The more spiral the incisions, which must be perfectly symmetrical, the quicker and less difficult the healing. Actually, because of the bridge of tissue in the surgical pattern, the cornea remains strong. It was much stronger with a disconnected hexagon than with a connected hexagon. By going past the apices, we were getting much greater results with the disconnected spiral hexagon.

With the six-incision spiral hexagon, I was able to correct up to five diopters of farsightedness, although the average result is two to three diopters.

In more than 300 of my own cases, to achieve good vision required more time than is required with radial keratotomy. With HK, it took approximately two to three months, with vision continuing to improve throughout the entire postoperative period.

As with RK, HK is a permanent surgical correction. There were postoperative complications similar to those of RK patients: glare and fluctuating vision, although less than RK patients experience.

In about a third of the patients in my study, induced astigmatism developed, a complication that was easily correctable by making flag, or "t," incisions on the cornea outside the hexagon. *Fig. 8-d.* Actually, the hexagonal pattern alone sometimes eliminated pre-existing astigmatism, but other times astigmatism was induced or increased. For the most part, however, induced astigmatism was regular (symmetrical).

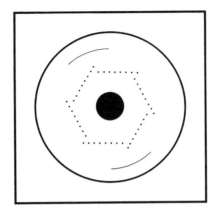

Fig. 8-d Grandon's disconnected spiral hexagon with flag, or "t" incisions

Three to four months after the hexagon was mostly healed, I was able to return to the eye and usually correct the astigmatism with "t" cuts outside the disconnected spiral hexagon pattern. My contributions to the HK procedure were twofold: Quantifying the ability to correct pre-existing or induced astigmatism following HK and quantifying the effect of disconnected spiral hexagonal surgery in the first place.

In one of the first articles published in an ophthalmology journal, I evaluated my study on hexagonal keratotomy. The article, "Hexagonal keratotomy safe, effective for primary hyperopia," appeared in *Ophthalmology Times* in September, 1993.

The article explained that I conducted a perspective evaluation of non-intersecting (disconnected), staggered spiral hexagonal keratotomy on 135 eyes. The mean patient age was 50 years, and the follow-up of the group ranged from three months to three years, with a mean of 10 months.

The article further stated that I was pleased with the success rate of the hexagonal procedure. The mean uncorrected acuity increased from 20/149 preoperatively to 20/50 postoperatively, while the incidence of 20/40 or better increased from 9% to 46%. These were very good results, and most of the patients themselves were very pleased with them.

Although other studies have reported problems with surgically induced irregular astigmatism, its occurrence was rare in my study, and it was correctable with topography analysis and accurate "t-cut" planning.

Emory University published a study showing complications after different types of HK. Many patient eyes underwent as many as nine operations. Also, the design and second procedure were different from what I did. There were cases of infection, scarring, and irregular astigmatism.

My completed study of disconnected spiral hexagonal keratotomy was published, and it basically showed the same results discussed above. As my experience grew, so did my patients' overall satisfaction. The complication rate was extremely low, and there have been no serious complications.

This was the only procedure to correct farsightedness that had a long history, good results, and publication in the best peer review journals. While I feel that it was an extremely important and accurate procedure, it was extremely difficult to perform and, today, it is rarely being done.

The problem is that other opthalmologists used other techniques. With the publication of my study, I had hoped more and more skilled surgeons would use my procedures and that they would gain more widespread acceptance. Unfortunately, that was not the case. Surgeons who used other techniques that they were not fully trained to perform occasionally had results that led to some complications.

Although hexagonal keratotomy is no longer being performed, there is hope for the farsighted. Hyperopic LASIK already shows promise in the correction of hyperopia. Also, phakic intraocular lenses are achieving good results in the correction of hyperopia.

Excimer Laser for correcting up to +6 diopters of hyperopia has been approved by the FDA for use in the United States.

Astigmatic keratotomy

Astigmatic keratotomy (AK), developed by Dr. Luis Ruiz of Mexico, is a variation of the surgery that corrects myopia and hyperopia.

Astigmatic keratotomy, which consists of making a number of flag, or "t," incisions on the surface of the cornea [*Fig. 8-e*], can be performed to correct astigmatism alone. The surgeon can also perform it at the same time he performs radial keratotomy. *Fig. 8-f.* With HK, astigmatic keratotomy requires two stages; HK is performed first, then AK is performed some time later.

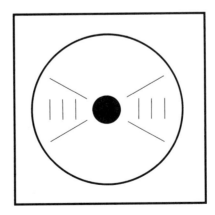

Fig. 8-e   Ruiz trapezoidal keratotomy for correction of astigmatism

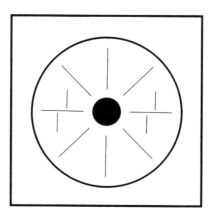

Fig. 8-f   Flag incision pattern used with radial incisions for correction of myopia and astigmatism

One modification I made in Ruiz's procedure, in my opinion, works better in certain situations. *Fig. 8-g.*

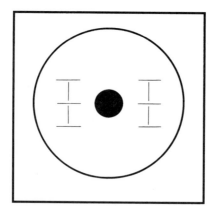

Fig. 8-g   Grandon modification of Ruiz procedure for correction of astigmatism alone

Dr. Spencer Thornton, a pioneer in the development of different astigmatic surgery design patterns, has used arcuate "t" incisions for astigmatism. It seems to improve the accuracy of "t" incisions and yield a more effective result. *Fig. 8-h.*

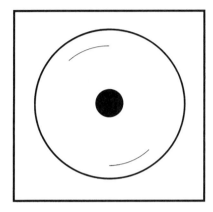

Fig. 8-h   Thornton's arcuate, or "t," incision pattern for astigmatism

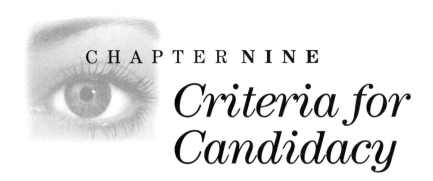

CHAPTER NINE
Criteria for Candidacy

The RK patient
Ophthalmologists involved in the ARK Study Group developed their own protocols, which dictated the guidelines of radial keratotomy procedures from patient selection to postoperative care. Part of my protocol that addressed patient selection serves as the basis for this chapter.

When a prospective patient telephones the Eye Surgery Institute in Dearborn, Michigan, to inquire about RK, the appointment secretary conducts a brief interview to determine if the individual will fit initial screening requirements with regard to age, the presence of myopia, and the absence of significant eye disease. If the individual passes this stage, the patient makes an appointment for a thorough examination.

Determining eligibility
To qualify for RK surgery, the following criteria must be present:

- The patient must have passed his or her 18th birthday.

- The patient must have two eyes correctable to about 20/40 vision or better.

- The degree of myopia must be at least -1 diopter (to be determined by one of the preoperative tests).

- There must be an absence of significant uncontrolled or rapidly progressive eye disease.

- Both myopia and astigmatism should be demonstrated to be relatively stable for a minimum of 18 months prior to RK surgery.

The degree of astigmatism, generally, will not be a limiting factor; however, higher degrees of astigmatism may require special surgical procedures. Transverse, or "flag," incisions can be made with the radial incisions for RK. For higher degrees of astigmatism, more transverse incisions can be made.

Myopic individuals with -3 diopters or less are generally considered to be good candidates for radial keratotomy, because their myopia is not severe and they can usually be corrected to good vision (20/40) or better.

People with -3 to -6 diopters fall into the mid-range of myopia and can usually be corrected to the point of not wearing corrective lenses for daily activities (20/40 or better).

Patients with -6 or more diopters are high myopes and, consequently, are usually more difficult to correct fully. Often the surgeon will have to use a technique known as *redeepening* to retrace the initial radial incisions and make them deeper. In other cases, the surgeon may opt to perform a second RK procedure at a later date to help the patient achieve the desired level of correction. Even with two operations, a complete correction may not result. [Again, with current LASIK technology, with -6 diopters or more, I prefer to do LASIK. Under unusual circumstances, I might do RK up to -8 diopters.]

Surgeons perform second procedures, known as touch-ups or *enhancements*, when the first operation yields an undercorrection. Many surgeons who do not have the advantage of computer software to guide the amount of surgery will undercorrect as a precautionary measure. Some of these surgeons are performing enhancements on as many as 50 to 60 percent of their RK patients, often returning to the eyes two or three times to get the desired correction.

In my own situation, my brother, Dr. Gary M. Grandon, and I developed outstanding computer software. Thanks to that software, I performed touch-ups on only about 15 percent of my RK patients, and those were usually high myopes or more difficult cases.

Back to the criteria for candidacy. The patient must be willing and mentally competent to receive adequate information regarding the indications, contraindications, and possible complications of the procedure. The patient must sign a detailed informed consent document prior to surgery (see Chapter 10).

Preoperative examinations

Preoperative patient examinations usually consist of one or two visits to the ophthalmologist to take a complete ophthalmic history and to accurately measure corneal curvature, thickness, and refractive error.

If contact lenses are worn, they must be removed and not used for 48 hours prior to the initial eye examination.

Preoperative examinations include the following:

- visual acuity

- keratometry (for corneal curvature)

- applanation tonometry (for eye pressure readings)

- ultrasound pachymetry (of utmost importance in determining the depth setting of the diamond knife)

- corneal diameter

- refraction with and without dilating eye drops, and

- corneal topography (a computer-assisted videokeratometer that gives extremely accurate keratometric readings and other corneal topography information; very helpful to the surgeon in planning surgery).

At the time of the complete examination, a history will be taken emphasizing the reason for the patient's desire to undergo RK surgery. This history will include vocational, avocational, general visual, and physiological reasons.

A history of past or present contact lens wearing experience will be obtained. A history of any current eye glare symptoms or problems in past ocular history, including ophthalmic surgical procedures, will be taken in detail. A medical history and a family ocular history will also be obtained.

Following the necessary examinations, the physician will interview the patient, clarifying and amplifying any pertinent historical points. The physician will then discuss with the patient the degree of stability of the patient's myopia and astigmatism, and the patient's estimated suitability for the surgery. The patient's reasons for desiring surgery will be discussed. If the patient is an unsatisfied current or past contact lens wearer, he will be informed that it may be possible with more current contact lenses to satisfy that patient's visual needs through contact lenses.

Dominant eye

There is general understanding that the response of the first eye to RK surgery (or refractive surgery of any type) is perhaps the most important predictor of the response of the second eye. It is important, therefore, for the surgeon to determine the non-dominant eye that should undergo RK surgery first. If the non-dominant eye is significantly less myopic, the ophthalmologist and the patient will decide which eye will undergo surgery first.

Finalizing patient selection

In most cases, the patient will have already read a patient information booklet regarding radial keratotomy. The physician will discuss with the patient any specific questions that require more detailed explanations or which are of particular concern to the patient.

The physician will provide the patient with information on his own statistical results and those of the range of myopia into which the patient falls. The patient will be told specifically that re-operation may be necessary and that overcorrection may occur at first and could be permanent, to some degree. (See Chapter 12 for information about overcorrection.)

The patient will be told that glasses may be necessary some or all of the time postoperatively. He can also expect to wear reading glasses after reaching approximately 45 years of age, just as he would if he had not had RK surgery.

There will be adequate opportunity for the patient to ask questions and receive answers in sufficient detail to inform him of the known and unknown aspects of RK surgery.

AK patient criteria
AK patient candidates must also pass a prescreening test to determine if he or she:

- is age 18 or older

- has two healthy eyes, and

- has no pre-existing corneal disease.

If a candidate has myopia and also has astigmatism, he should be able to qualify for refractive surgery to correct either a myopia-astigmatism combination or astigmatism by itself, providing the candidate has met the prescreening criteria.

Upon meeting the prescreening requirements, astigmatic candidates undergo the same preoperative examinations that the myopic candidate experiences.

LASIK patient criteria
In addition to the criteria mentioned above for AK surgery, there is evolving technology that enables the patient and surgeon to select the best procedure to correct astigmatism, with or without myopia. The guidelines, with regard to the degree of myopia, for choosing RK or LASIK, are as follows:

-3 and fewer diopters of myopia — RK surgery
    (or LASIK, if wanted)
-3 to -6 diopters — either RK or LASIK (price is an issue)
-6 and more diopters — LASIK.

RK is still a good procedure for lower degrees of myopia and astigmatism. LASIK can correct astigmatism with or without myopia; in fact, we can correct higher degrees of astigmatism with LASIK than with RK.

CHAPTER **TEN**

Informed Consent –
Making an Educated Decision

Radial keratotomy
Prior to scheduling radial keratotomy surgery, the patient should carefully study the surgeon's informed consent on the procedure in order to make an educated decision. The physician should answer all questions satisfactorily before the patient signs the informed consent.

A good informed consent for radial keratotomy should offer information about alternative treatments of myopia; namely, those mentioned in Chapter 5 of this book.

At clinics, such as the Eye Surgery Institute of Dearborn, where ongoing studies of radial keratotomy have been conducted, the informed consent explains the conditions of the study and the patient's obligations to participate in it, should the patient choose to do so.

A good informed consent should offer the following information, which a patient should declare he or she understands before signing it.

- *This particular surgery consists of making a number of cuts (8 to 16 or more) on the surface of the cornea of my eye. The surgeon makes these cuts in order to effect the flattening of the central portion of my cornea or to change astigmatism. By so doing, my vision may be improved even to the point of not wearing glasses.*

- *The results of surgery in my case cannot be guaranteed.*

- *As a result of the surgery, it is possible that my vision may be made worse. This could happen as a result of infection that could not be controlled with antibiotics or other means, in which case it may be possible that the eye could be lost. This could also occur due to irregular healing of the incisions such that the corneal surface would be distorted. I understand that, in that case, it may be necessary for me to wear a contact lens to effect useful vision and that there is a possibility that this may not restore useful vision.*

  It is also possible that the results of surgery may not be obtained and that, at a later date, it may become necessary to have further treatment that may include additional surgery.

- *I understand that if I presently wear bifocals or reading glasses, I will still need a reading glass prescription after having radial keratotomy.*

- *I understand that glare with night driving, halos around headlights, and star-shaped figures around lights occur after surgery. Usually these conditions go away with time. However, it is possible that they can persist indefinitely.*

- *Fluctuating vision [different vision at different times of day] occurs after surgery. This condition usually disappears with time. However, it may persist to some degree indefinitely.*

- *Double vision may occur between operations (before the second eye is operated on) because of the different image size in the first eye that has had surgery, compared to the second eye that has not had surgery and that still requires the use of an eyeglass. If the second eye uses a contact lens instead of an eyeglass, the double vision usually goes away. If, for any reason, the second eye does not undergo surgery and is not fitted with a contact lens, double vision with glasses may persist and cause vision problems. This condition is usually worse in cases of higher myopia.*

- *An undercorrection or overcorrection can occur. If an undercorrection occurs, usually the ophthalmologist can perform more surgery at a later date. If an overcorrection occurs, radial keratotomy cannot correct it, but there is another surgical procedure that can correct it.*

- *After surgery, if needed for complete correction, the patient can usually wear contact lenses successfully. However, in some cases, contact lenses might not be able to be successfully worn. In any case, the patient cannot have a contact lens fitting until after a waiting period of many months.*

- *Following surgery, there usually are no scars, and with the naked eye under normal lighting conditions, rarely will anyone be able to detect that surgery has been performed. Occasionally, with very close observation, lines might be visible.*

The informed consent continues:

> *I understand that the longest follow-up of radial keratotomy patients has been 25 years in the Soviet Union and 17 years in the United States. I also understand that unforeseen complications such as irregularity or clouding may occur at a later date.*

> **Complications of surgery in general**

> *As with all types of surgery, there is a possibility of other complications. The proper informed consent for radial keratotomy should state that complications might include anesthetics (including local anesthetics given for eye surgery), drug reactions or other factors that may involve other parts of the patient's body. It is impossible to state every complication that may occur as a result of any surgery, so the list of complications in an informed consent will be incomplete.*

The informed consent continues:

> *The basic procedures of radial keratotomy, the advantages and disadvantages, risks, and possible complications of this procedure and alternative treatments of nearsightedness have been explained to me by the ophthalmologist. Although it is impossible for the physician to inform me of every possible complication that may occur, he has answered all my questions to my satisfaction.*

> *I understand that performing this surgery on my eye is part of a clinical investigation. Periodic visits to the ophthalmologist will be required for at least one year to assess the results of the operation, and an annual follow-up of five years will be requested.*

I give permission for medical data concerning my operation and subsequent treatment to be released to investigators and responsible authorities demonstrating a "need to know" for the clinical study described.

I understand that I may withdraw from the clinical study at any time without jeopardizing my future medical care.

I acknowledge that the physician has not provided information inconsistent with any statements in this informed consent document.

Signing this informed consent for radial keratotomy surgery indicates that I have read this document (or someone has read it to me). I fully understand and accept the possible risks, complications, and benefits that can result from the surgery.

If the ophthalmologist is participating in an ongoing clinical study, the informed consent should provide a space where the patient can indicate that he or she is willing to participate in the study. A simple box for checking "yes" or "no" box is sufficient. The patient then signs the informed consent. A witness and the physician should also sign the document.

After the patient signs the informed consent, he schedules a convenient time for radial keratotomy surgery.

Astigmatic keratotomy

The informed consent for radial keratotomy covers all the necessary information required for informing a patient who plans to undergo refractive surgery for the correction of astigmatism. No separate informed consent is necessary.

The surgeon should explain a few additional points, however. Astigmatic keratotomy can take a long time to produce good results.

It should also be noted that if, in doing astigmatic keratotomy, the surgeon shifts astigmatism to another axis and, therefore, overcorrects, it is possible to re-suture (add more "t" or arcuate "t" incisions) and correct the problem.

LASIK

The informed consent for LASIK notes that eyeglasses and contact lenses are the most common method of correcting nearsightedness, farsightedness, and astigmatism. When tolerated well, they are likely to be a good alternative to LASIK surgery. Refractive surgery is continually evolving and other refractive procedures may be available as an alternative to LASIK.

It goes on to say that LASIK permanently changes the shape of the cornea. The surgery is performed under a topical anesthetic (drops in the eye). The procedure involves folding back a thin layer of corneal tissue (corneal flap) and then removing a thin layer of corneal tissue with the light from an Excimer laser. After removal, the surgeon replaces the flap and bonds it back into place without the need for stitches. The result of removing thin layers of tissue causes the center of the cornea to flatten in the case of nearsightedness, or steepen in the case of farsightedness, or become more rounded in the case of astigmatism, which changes the focusing power of the cornea. Although the goal of LASIK is to improve vision to the point of removing the patient's dependency on glasses or contact lenses or to the point of allowing him or her to wear thinner (weaker) glasses, this result is not guaranteed.

The patient should also understand that LASIK will not prevent him from developing naturally-occurring eye problems such as glaucoma, cataracts, retinal degeneration or detachment. After the procedure, the patient should avoid rubbing the eye. Eyes may be more susceptible to traumatic injury after LASIK (at least in the early healing phase), and protective eye wear is recommended for all contact and racquet sports where a direct blow to the eye could occur. Also, LASIK does not correct the condition known as presbyopia (or aging of the eye) that occurs to most people around the age of 40, possibly requiring them to wear reading glasses for close-up work. People over 40 who have had their nearsightedness corrected may find that they need reading glasses for clear, close vision.

The informed consent lists the potential risks of LASIK, including:

1. LOSS OF VISION. LASIK surgery can possibly cause loss of vision or loss of best corrected vision. This can be due to infection or irregular scarring or other causes, and unless successfully controlled by antibiotics, steroids, or other necessary treatment, could even cause loss of the infected eye. Vision loss can be due to the cornea healing irregularly that could add astigmatism and make wearing glasses or contact lenses necessary, and useful vision could be lost. It is also possible that the patient may not be able to successfully wear contacts after LASIK.

2. VISUAL SIDE EFFECTS. Other complications and conditions that can occur with LASIK include: anisometropia (difference in power between the two eyes); aniseikonia (difference in image size between the two eyes); double vision; hazy vision; fluctuating vision during the day and from day to day; increased sensitivity to light which may

be incapacitating for some time and may not completely go away; glare, and halos around lights that may not completely go away. Some of these conditions may affect the patient's ability to drive and judge distances. Driving should be done only when he is certain his vision is adequate.

3. OVERCORRECTION AND UNDERCORRECTION: It may be that LASIK surgery will not give the patient the result he desires. Many procedures result in the eye being undercorrected, in which case it may be possible or necessary to have additional surgery to fine-tune or enhance the initial result. These results cannot be guaranteed. It is also possible that the eye may be overcorrected to the point of remaining farsighted. It is also possible that the initial results could regress over time. In some, but not all cases, retreatment could be considered.

4. OTHER RISKS: Additional reported complications include: corneal ulcer formation; endothelial cell loss; epithelial healing defects; ptosis (droopy eye lid); corneal swelling; retinal detachment; and hemorrhage. Complications could also arise requiring further corrective procedures, including either a partial (lamellar) or full thickness corneal transplant using a donor cornea. These complications include: loss of corneal disc; damage to the corneal disc; disc decentration; and progressive corneal thinning (extasia). Sutures may also be required that could induce astigmatism. There are also potential complications due to anesthesia and medications that may involve other parts of the patient's body. It is also possible that the microkeratome or the Excimer laser could malfunction and the procedure be stopped. Since it is impossible to state all potential risks of any surgery, this informed consent is incomplete.

5. FUTURE COMPLICATIONS: The patient should also be aware that there are other complications that could occur that have not been reported before the creation of this informed consent, as LASIK surgery has been performed only since the early 1990s, and longer term results may reveal additional risks and complications.

6. LASIK is considered an "off label" use of an approved medical device. Off label usage of FDA-approved devices and medications are commonly practiced by physicians without interference from the FDA and allows physicians to practice medicine in a manner they feel most beneficial to their patients.

The LASIK informed consent concludes with postoperative instructions, as follows:

After LASIK surgery, the patient will be given medications and instructions to help prevent infection and control healing. It is imperative that he follow ALL instructions exactly as they are given to him. It is also imperative that all follow-up visits be kept as directed.

The patient is then given the opportunity, providing his questions have been answered and he understands potential risks of LASIK, to sign the consent form for surgery.

CHAPTER ELEVEN
Refractive Surgery (RK & AK) Today –
The Operations

Preoperative preparations

The steps leading to the actual surgery in RK and AK are identical. The only differences become apparent during surgery itself.

Surgeons perform refractive surgery in a clinic or hospital on an outpatient basis. At the Eye Surgery Institute of Dearborn, for example, patients generally arrive an hour and a half before surgery and usually leave a half hour or so following the operation.

In the hour immediately preceding surgery, the patient receives eye drops and often some medications to help him relax. At this time, the surgeon may take final measurements of the cornea.

When the patient arrives in the operating room, he lies down on the operating table. The eye that will undergo surgery receives surgical scrubs from the ophthalmic technologist. The patient may then be draped appropriately for ophthalmic surgery.

A special eye drape exposing only the eye undergoing surgery is loosely placed over the patient's face, and a topical anesthetic is administered. The drops of 4% xylocaine, packaged in individual sterile vials, sting a little when applied, but they are necessary to numb the cornea so the patient will not feel anything during surgery.

A tiny wire lid speculum holds open the eye, preventing the patient from closing his eye during surgery. *Fig. 11-a.*

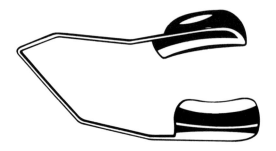

Fig. 11-a   The lid speculum holds the eye open during surgery.

The surgeon carefully checks the instruments to make certain that the length, depth and selection of incisions will be precisely maintained. He checks the clear zone marker to make sure it corresponds to the patient's needs (for myopia and/or astigmatism). In radial keratotomy, the smaller clear zone renders the larger correction. Three millimeters is considered a small clear zone.

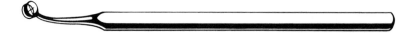

Fig. 11-b   The clear zone market determines the amount of correction.

The corneal marker enables the surgeon to mark where he will make the incisions for radial keratotomy, as well as for correcting astigmatism. *Fig. 11-c.*

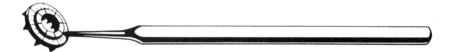

Fig. 11-c The Grandon corneal market indicates where the surgeon will make the incisions.

Following the corneal marking, the surgeon applies a few drops of fluorescein, a dye, to more clearly define where he will make the incisions.

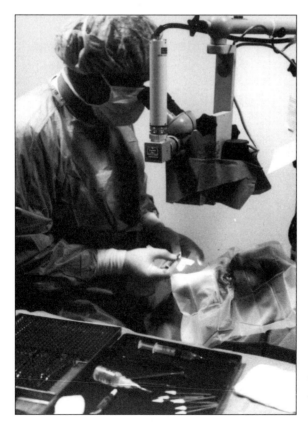

Dr. Grandon performing radial keratotomy

The operation

The surgeon operates while looking through a high-powered surgical microscope. He uses a diamond-tipped knife with a micrometer handle that enables him to adjust the blade for depth on incision and lock it in place. He makes the prescribed number of incisions on the surface of the cornea, leaving the clear zone in the center untouched.

There are different surgical patterns involved in the three types of refractive procedures: radial for RK and "t" or arcuate "t" for AK.

In radial keratotomy, the surgeon makes from 6 to 16 incisions, allowing the central part of the cornea to flatten. Flattening the cornea permits full or partial correction. *Fig. 11-d* and *Fig. 11-e*.

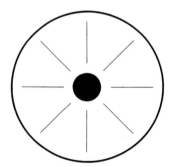

Fig. 11-d 8-incision RK surgery pattern

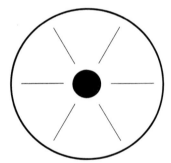

Fig. 11-e 6-incision RK surgery pattern

There are two principal differences in how to perform radial keratotomy. One is the Soviet technique, in which the surgeon makes radial incisions from outside in toward the optical zone. In the American technique, which I use, the incisions go from the outer edge of the optical zone out toward the edge of the cornea.

Fyodorov developed the Soviet technique, of course, because he thought he could achieve a better result and, with a metal blade he may have done so. Bores developed the American technique that, I believe, with the diamond knife, is infinitely safer. The Soviet technique is dangerous for two reasons: (1) the surgeon can cut through the visual axis, and (2) the cornea gets thinner towards the middle, possibly resulting in a larger perforation. A larger perforation can cause serious problems, such as a higher risk for infection that can lead to serious complications.

The surgeon secures the eyeball with a very small forceps while he makes the incisions. During the procedure, the patient feels only slight pressure on the eye.

At the completion of surgery, the incisions are carefully counted to make sure the proper number has been made. An incision depth gauge checks the depths of the incisions. Each incision is irrigated with a saline solution, then the eye is given antibiotic eye drops. A patch is then placed over the eye.

The patient proceeds to a postoperative room, where the surgeon instructs him to keep the patch on for at least an hour and to administer the prescribed eye drops.

RK for high myopes

In the early days of radial keratotomy, individuals with high degrees of myopia (more than -6 diopters) were not considered good candidates for this operation. However, RK for higher myopia often gave very good results. Now, with newer technology, these techniques give even better results statistically.

In my own experience, however, good results were achieved with high myopes. Many of my patients who had -8, -9 or more diopters of myopia achieved complete correction, often without redeepening or two separate operations. In redeepening, the surgeon retraces the first radial incisions in the periphery, where the cornea is deeper, with increased diamond depth at the time of the initial operation. This procedure gave added result for high myopes. I published the first paper on redeepening four or five years ago in the *American Journal of Cataract and Refractive Surgery,* and it showed that redeepening gave increased results.

If the high myope did not achieve a sufficient correction, he may have undergone a second procedure (an enhancement) for added results. In this procedure, either four or eight incisions (usually four) were added between the original incisions.

To date, the results of radial keratotomy for higher myopes (-6 diopters and above) have been good for patients who were once totally dependent on very thick corrective lenses. RK results for the low and mid-range myopia groups, on a statistical basis, are better. If glasses are still needed, they are not as thick and cumbersome as they once were, and the patient enjoys substantially improved vision without glasses.

It is still possible that some individuals are too myopic for RK. In a young person, about -8 is the most that can usually be corrected, while a person 40 to 50 years of age can achieve a correction of -9 or more diopters of myopia. If someone has very high myopia and can wear contact lenses, I would not perform radial keratotomy on that person.

The above is of historical interest. Today, for patients with over -6.0D myopia, LASIK is recommended. Phakic intraocular lenses are also being developed and tested in this area. In certain parts of the world, RK may still be done for high myopes, and the results, as shown above, can be quite good.

RK for myopes with astigmatism

Many people who are myopic also have some degree of astigmatism, a condition that causes blurring of objects in space. Patients with high degrees of astigmatism welcome the trapezoidal keratotomy, or the Ruiz procedure, which can correct eight or nine diopters of astigmatism. The Mexican ophthalmologist, Dr. Luis Ruiz, developed this procedure. The design calls for radial incisions with three or four transverse incisions.

For people with both myopia and astigmatism, various designs of elliptical clear zones combined with tangential or flag incisions can be used to correct the aspherosity of the cornea (make it spherical).

LASIK can also correct astigmatism, even high astigmatism, probably even better than with AK.

CHAPTER TWELVE

Post-Op Complications, Care, and Expectations

Following RK surgery, the physician gives the patient a prescription for antibiotic eye drops, cautions him to rest the eye until the patch is removed, and to wear sunglasses in bright light.

The operated eye will remain a little sensitive for a few days, until the end of the first week, when sight is often significantly improved. At this time, the patient may schedule surgery for the second eye, if the first procedure was radial keratotomy. Both eyes almost never undergo surgery at the same time. The surgical design on the second eye depends on the result of the first eye, because we know how it has healed. We have achieved a lower re-operation rate by doing one eye at a time.

During the early postoperative period, most patients can expect to experience some irritation. It is similar to the sensation when a foreign body, such as a grain of sand, is in the eye.

In the case of postoperative RK, the eye will usually be farsighted for the first week or two, then that condition regresses as the corrected vision begins to stabilize. The patient often notices glare, star-shaped figures around headlights, and some fluctuating vision. All these postoperative conditions, which are normal (even for cases following other kinds of refractive surgery), should be no cause for alarm, and usually improve with time.

During this period, the physician may impose some or all of the following restrictions:

- *Do not wear eye makeup for 10 days following surgery.*

- *Do not swim for 10 days following surgery.*

- *Do not drive on the day of surgery nor while taking strong pain medications, if prescribed.*

- *Wear safety glasses when playing tennis, racquetball, etc.*

- *Wear a seat belt when driving or riding as a passenger.*

- *Do not wear contact lenses for six months after surgery on the eye or eyes that have undergone surgery.*

- *Wear sunglasses in bright light immediately after surgery.*

- *Since marijuana causes changes in eye pressure, it therefore should not be used throughout the healing period.*

Otherwise, the patient may shampoo immediately after surgery, do any strenuous exercise, or work immediately after the surgery.

Postoperative examinations

Postoperative examinations are conducted on the first post-op day and at regular intervals as determined by the patient's needs. At the Eye Surgery Institute of Dearborn, for instance, we conducted two- to three-week, three-month, and yearly examinations to gather data for my ongoing study of radial keratotomy. Each postop examination includes a history, as well as refraction and visual acuity tests.

After the healing is complete, the cornea will have taken on a new shape. That shape will be quite permanent. As Fyodorov once said, "It is like changing the shape of your nose. Once the cornea is changed, it is permanent. Over the past several years, no reversion to its previous shape has been experienced."

Complications

Performed by an expert microsurgeon, the complication rate for RK is extremely low and continues to diminish.

In addition to some of the postoperative conditions mentioned earlier in this chapter, which may persist beyond the normal healing period, the most common complications of RK are:

- *overcorrection, which now can be helped by a different surgical procedure. The last thing a nearsighted person wants is an overcorrection, to be made farsighted. Fortunately, if overcorrection occurs, it is sometimes possible to reverse it. The procedure requires the surgeon to reopen the radial incisions, remove the collagen material from the incisions, and put in four sutures (stitches), which will remain for a year or more. Also, in recent months, ALK has been successful in treating overcorrected RKs. (This is still controversial.) New combinations of medications can often reverse overcorrection. More recently, LASIK over RK has been able to achieve good results in either reducing or eliminating RK over-corrections. We must wait one year for healing before we can perform LASIK to correct the overcorrection.*

- *undercorrection, which can be remedied by a second RK procedure, known as a touch-up or an enhancement, at a later date. Dr. Dennis Shepard of California has also introduced a non-surgical technique that helps undercorrected patients achieve a better result. We refer to the technique as **knuckling**. If a patient is undercorrected at two or more weeks postop, he takes steroid eye drops for six weeks to perhaps gain one diopter of a better result. He may pick up another diopter of result if he presses gently on his eye for 20 seconds four times a day. I have recommended knuckling to my patients for the past three years, and have found the results to be encouraging.*

Expectations

No matter how much one reads about refractive surgery beforehand or understands the risks, possible complications, and postoperative care of such surgery, one always hopes for a good result. The danger is in expecting more than the surgeon can deliver. Each human heals differently, responds to medications and surgery differently, and consequently achieves a result compatible with his own unique physiological make-up. Not everyone, therefore, will achieve 20/20 vision, so it is unrealistic to expect that result, no matter how skilled the surgeon. (Most people who achieve 20/30 or 20/40 wear glasses. In Michigan, one needs 20/40 uncorrected vision in one eye to get an unrestricted driver's license.) By the way, it is not necessary to achieve 20/20 uncorrected vision to lead a full and happy life.

What a refractive surgery patient can expect is a set of postoperative feelings, sensations, and symptoms in common with most other refractive surgery patients.

During surgery, with relaxing medications at work and a topical anesthetic doing its job to numb the cornea, the patient will feel no pain. He will feel only a slight amount of pressure as the surgeon makes the incisions. The patient will see only the bright white light of the microscope. He may chat with the surgeon, and before he knows it, the surgery is finished and he is ready to leave the operating room.

After surgery, depending on his own pain threshold, he can expect to feel some discomfort or pain (again, depending on his definition) as the effects of the anesthetic and medications diminish. People with a low tolerance for pain might describe the postoperative period as a personal horror, having them seek the shelter of their own bed for a couple of days. Individuals with high pain thresholds, on the other hand, often find the discomfort so inconsequential that they return to work the same day or the day after surgery.

Also, following surgery, patients can expect to experience glare, fluctuating vision, and star-shaped figures around lights, especially around headlights during night driving. Usually these occurrences will improve with time but may persist indefinitely. These postop events are normal, as we have stated in the informed consent in Chapter 10. Some patients can expect to wait longer for improved vision, sometimes not seeing better for two or three days or more, while other patients see great improvement when they remove the eye patch.

At any rate, these are some of the normal situations that most refractive surgery patients can expect to experience.

Criteria for re-operations
Even with our sophisticated computer software that dictates guidelines for RK and AK surgery, we still face the fact that we are dealing with a biological system, after all. Everyone

heals differently. The nature of collagen varies from one individual to another. Therefore, there will probably always be a need for touch-up procedures.

Reoperations with radial keratotomy patients are usually considered only for the following reasons: when the results obtained do not meet the patient's satisfaction, when uncorrected visual acuity is less than the patient wants, and where there is clear opportunity to add further incisions or reduce the size of the clear zone.

According to my own experience, I do not perform a re-operation until at least three months have passed. If I reoperate, I do not usually redeepen any incisions that I have already made.

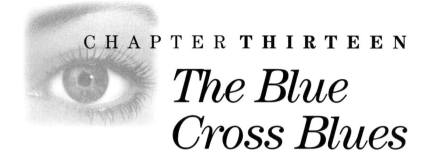

CHAPTER THIRTEEN
The Blue Cross Blues

Ability to pay for medical care or surgical treatment has always been a primary consideration. Today, with the health care issue at center stage throughout the country, it has taken on even greater significance.

In 1985 and early 1986, two of my RK patients, Arthur Sumeracki and Robert Cieslik, underwent radial keratotomy to correct severe myopia. Both patients had received assurances from Blue Cross/Blue Shield of Michigan that radial keratotomy was a covered benefit. In Sumeracki's case, BCBSM paid $920 for each operation, but on December 18, 1986, they rejected his claim and demanded a refund of the amounts paid.

In Cieslik's case, BCBSM paid the invoice submitted after the first RK surgery, but rejected the invoice submitted after the second surgery.

BCBSM maintained that it was correct and not in violation of state law in denying benefits, because radial keratotomy was not a generally accepted operative and cutting procedure in 1985.

Radial keratotomy as a surgical procedure was first performed in the United States in 1978. Both the Michigan Ophthalmology Society and the American Academy of Ophthalmology classified RK as experimental. BCBSM relied upon this classification by the professional organizations in determining that the surgical procedure was experimental and thus not a generally accepted procedure.

As early as 1983, however, the American Academy of Ophthalmology changed the classification of radial keratotomy from experimental to investigational. BCBSM has determined that at least some surgical procedures that are investigational are generally accepted procedures.

In December of 1984, the Michigan Ophthalmology Society determined that radial keratotomy was no longer experimental. The Michigan Ophthalmology Society sent a letter to BCBSM informing it of this determination. In part, pertinent to the issue at hand, the letter said:

Please let the record show that the Michigan Ophthalmology Society has re-evaluated radial keratotomy and retracted the previous statement tagging the technique "experimental." Although it had not received the Society's complete blessing, we no longer label it "experimental."

Subsequent correspondence from the Michigan Ophthalmology Society shows that removing radial keratotomy from the experimental category meant that the Society regarded it as a generally accepted procedure. These 1986 documents are important to an understanding of the significance of the December 1984 determination by the Michigan Ophthalmology Society. They are also pertinent, because BCBSM made its determination to recoup payments in 1986.

The Michigan Ophthalmology Society, in a letter to BCBSM dated January 31, 1985, plainly advised that the Society no longer considered radial keratotomy surgery to be experimental. On February 20, 1986, John W. Cowden, M.D., of the Kresge Eye Institute in Detroit, Michigan, wrote to BCBSM. On behalf of the Michigan Ophthalmology Society, he advised that radial keratotomy was an established procedure that had been investigated for more than six years and was found to be safe and effective. On May 21, 1986, Cowden again advised BCBSM on a form provided by them that radial keratotomy surgery was not an experimental procedure and was generally used by the professional community.

Setting a precedent

On behalf of my patients, Sumeracki and Cieslik, as well as others whose claims had been rejected but who were not part of the initial suit, I sued Blue Cross/Blue Shield of Michigan. Class action lawsuits are difficult to undertake in Michigan, and individuals cannot afford to take on a giant like BCBSM. Therefore, I decided that we would enable them to do what they could not afford to do. Most of my patients are young and healthy individuals who have not utilized their health insurance. It seemed, therefore, particularly unfair to me that BCBSM would reject their claims.

The prestigious law firm of Bellamy and Gilchrist, P.C., in Detroit, was retained for the suit against the Blues giant, and Michael S. Cafferty became the attorney of record for Sumeracki and Cieslik. Cafferty handled the case brilliantly, as the result indicates.

On January 30, 1991, D. A. D'Annunzio, Michigan's Acting Commissioner of Insurance, handed down a ruling that BCBSM be required to honor patient claims for radial keratotomy surgery. We had scored a landmark victory over the Blues of Michigan! The ruling stated that in 1985, "radial keratotomy was a generally accepted procedure" and, therefore, BCBSM must honor claims for it.

The decision was issued after a full trial was held before Administrative Law Judge, the Honorable Edward Rogers, on behalf of Arthur Sumeracki and Robert Cieslik who, upon rejection by BCBSM, had filed complaints with the Insurance Bureau.

After the hearing, which lasted several days and included the testimony of several witnesses, Rogers ruled that BCBSM incorrectly labeled the procedure "experimental" and wrongfully rejected the claims. The earliest surgery involved in the case was performed in 1985. Rogers ruled that the evidence supported a finding that the surgery was not experimental when it was performed on either patient.

After Rogers' decision, BCBSM appealed the decision to the Insurance Commissioner who, in large part, upheld Rogers' conclusions. After reviewing the record of the trial, D'Annunzio ruled that BCBSM "did not conduct a reasonable investigation" of radial keratotomy prior to rejecting the claims.

In particular, D'Annunzio noted that BCBSM violated the law because it failed to "take into account the views of professional societies, especially those of the Michigan Ophthalmology Society, that radial keratotomy was no longer regarded as experimental as of December 1984." D'Annunzio noted that in 1985, "radial keratotomy was a generally accepted procedure." As a remedy, he ruled that BCBSM should pay the claims and "cease and desist" from further violation of the law.

On October 21, 1991, we scored a precedent-setting victory for radial keratotomy. The Honorable Lawrence Glazer, Ingham County [Michigan] Circuit Court Judge, after reviewing appellate briefs, stated that he would affirm the earlier decision of the Michigan Insurance Commission requiring BCBSM to pay claims for radial keratotomy.

In so ruling, Glazer said there was more than sufficient evidence that RK was a generally accepted procedure and that Blue Cross should pay. Shortly afterward, Glazer signed the order dismissing the Blues' appeal.

In the November 1, 1992, issue of its publication, *The Record*, BCBSM stated that it would pay for radial keratotomy. The average cost for this extremely delicate surgery is $1,200 to $1,500 per eye. Blue Cross was expected to pay only $425 per eye. [Now they are paying closer to $500 per eye.] "That amount is small," I said at the time, "but it's a start. Most radial keratotomy patients are young and healthy individuals who have not utilized their health insurance, so it was unfair when Blue Cross paid nothing. At least now, these patients will get some help."

With dismissal of the Blues' appeal, Michigan became the first state in the nation to force Blue Cross to pay claims for RK surgery.

The precedent-setting case carries national import. Blue Cross, in the past, has tried not to pay for new procedures. This case should make it easier for patients who have undergone other types of new procedures to take action against Blue Cross or other insurance carriers and also emerge victorious. It should also help other states to take appropriate action to make Blue Cross pay for RK and for other types of new surgery.

[At this time, Blue Cross, while paying for part of RK, is not paying for LASIK. Some other insurances have been paying some of the expenses of LASIK, but recently some of them have ceased doing that.]

CHAPTER FOURTEEN

Looking to Lasers –
The Excimer and Holmium Lasers

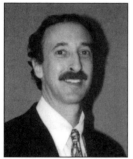

The section of Chapter 14 that discusses the Excimer Laser was contributed by Alan Spigelman, M.D., Michigan. Board certified, Dr. Spigelman served as the principal investigator for Sinai Hospital (Detroit) — FDA Excimer Laser Trials, 1991-1997.

Alan Spigelman, M.D.

The Excimer Laser

The Excimer Laser [*Fig. 14-a* and *Fig. 14-b*] was developed as an industrial laser in the late 1970s.

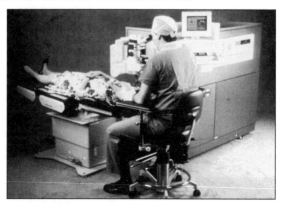

Fig. 14-a   VISX STAR Excimer Laser System

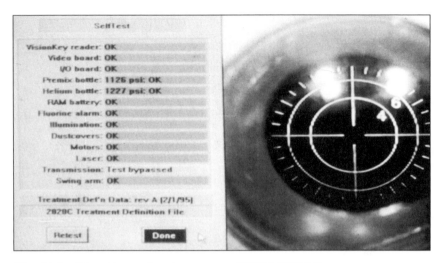

Fig. 14-b   View through microscope of VISX STAR Laser

In 1983, Drs. S. L. Trokel and R. Srinivasan noted that it may be used within a biological tissue. They were able to demonstrate that this laser could remove very precise amounts of tissue with each pulse. In fact, it removes approximately .025mm of tissue with a single application. This fact enabled researchers to manipulate the cornea to effect different refractive changes within the eye. The Excimer Laser can remove tissue without damaging adjacent structures. *Fig. 14-c. Figure 14-d* shows the Excimer Laser etching notches in a human hair.

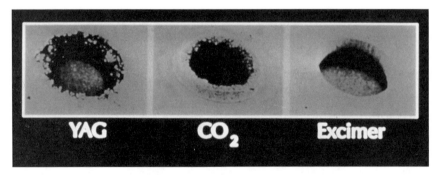

Fig. 14-c   YAG, CO_2, and Excimer ablation of plastic, demonstrating the smooth ablation characteristics of the Excimer laser

CHAPTER FOURTEEN LOOKING TO LASERS – THE EXCIMER AND HOLMIUM LASERS

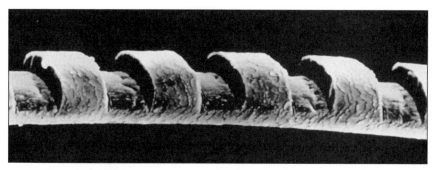

Fig. 14-d   The Excimer Laser etching notches in a human hair.

At this time, the Excimer Laser is under FDA study here in the United States. The first study that has already been completed is a therapeutic protocol. Within therapeutic protocols, people with scars in the cornea are treated. The data from this study shows that the Excimer Laser is indeed able to remove superficial scars from the cornea with preservation of good visual acuity. The FDA has now also approved Excimer Laser treatment from -1.00 to -12.00 diopters of myopia with up to 4.0 diopters of astigmatism. Treatment of hyperopia (farsightedness) is currently under investigation.

The next set of studies has to deal with low amounts of nearsightedness; that is, myopia up to -6 diopters. This encompasses the vast majority of patients who may be interested in refractive surgery. This study is now in Phase 3 of testing, which means all the patients have been lasered, and we are now collecting data to be submitted to the FDA. Approval of this technology will come probably within the next two to five years.

Additional studies that are now ongoing include high myopia. This study includes patients who have -6 to -12 diopters of myopia. This treatment is now in Phase 2 of trials, and early results have been quite encouraging. This study will probably be approved by the FDA within four to six years.

There are additional protocols evaluating higher amounts of nearsightedness. Correction of farsightedness is now being investigated. These studies are both in the very early phase of investigation; the results are too early to make any specific comments about them.

The Excimer Laser patient

A patient who is scheduled to undergo an Excimer Laser photorefractive keratoplasty arrives 20 to 30 minutes prior to the procedure. He is then given some oral Valium, if he is feeling nervous about the situation. After again discussing the overall procedure and what he can expect, the patient is brought to the laser suite. Once there, the surgeon discusses with him what will be accomplished. The patient's main goal during the laser treatment is to continue to fixate on a small flashing red light. If the patient is fixating on the appropriate spot, the surgeon knows that the laser beam is aligned properly. During the procedure, the surgeon continuously monitors the patient's eye under high magnification to ensure that it is indeed appropriately positioned.

Prior to having the patient seated at the laser, the computer that actually directs the laser throughout the procedure has been pre-programmed. The patient's preoperative refraction, which is an indication of the amount of nearsightedness and astigmatism to be corrected, has been entered into the laser as has additional data about the patient. Based on this data, the computer that calculates how much of an ablation is to be carried out, and it will also monitor the laser throughout the procedure to be sure that it is, in fact, achieved.

The patient is then seated at the laser, and an eye shield is placed over the unoperated eye. This is to prevent visual distractions from occurring during the laser procedure. The patient is then placed under the laser, and a topical anesthetic eye drop is applied to the eye. Once two sets of topical anes-

CHAPTER FOURTEEN   LOOKING TO LASERS – THE EXCIMER AND HOLMIUM LASERS

thetic have been placed into the eye, a lid speculum is attached. At this point, the patient is asked to fixate on the flashing red light. A 7mm optical zone marker that could also be used in radial keratotomy is centered over this visual axis and an imprint is made into the epithelium. A merocel sponge, cut to 6mm and soaked in topical Tetracaine, is applied to the cornea and left in place for one minute. The goal of this action is to soften the epithelial adhesions to the underlying cornea. The epithelium, which is the top layer of the eye, much like the top layer of your skin, will be removed by the surgeon manually prior to using the laser.

After the merocel sponge has been left in place for one minute, it is removed. Using a blunt, spatulated instrument, the superficial epithelium is scraped from its underlying attachments. This part of the process generally takes two to three minutes. After this process has been completed, the surgeon inspects the surface to ensure that it is absolutely smooth. At times, a small amount of fluid is applied to the cornea to ensure it is in the right hydration state prior to applying the laser.

Next, the light within the laser microscope is turned down so that the flashing fixation light can be more easily visualized by the patient. The patient is then instructed not to be startled when the laser starts up, as it is a fairly loud machine while it is working.

The patient is then encouraged to continuously watch the flashing red light throughout the procedure. As mentioned earlier, the surgeon continuously monitors the fixation of the patient's eye.

The surgeon is then able to depress the foot pedal, which engages the laser. If, at any time, the patient's eye moves, the laser can be stopped immediately by removing the foot from the laser foot pedal. The entire lasering procedure takes anywhere from 20 to 120 seconds, depending on the amount of nearsightedness. Most patients will probably be lasered within 20 to 40 seconds.

Once the procedure has been completed, a bandage contact lens is applied to the eye, as well as some topical medications, to keep the eye comfortable. The patient is then given postoperative pain medications and eye drops to use while at home.

In the early postoperative period, the patient can certainly experience discomfort. The application of the bandage contact lens helps to decrease the discomfort, as do the topical anti-inflammatory eye drops. The patient is also given some type of pain medication and is asked to use it liberally. Usually within three or four days, the top layer, which has been scraped, has healed. At this time, the eye feels normal.

The visual acuity is not improved until this top layer has healed and smoothed itself out. Usually this process takes anywhere from one to two weeks. If the patient has a lower amount of nearsightedness, usually at this time the vision has returned and is quite good. However, in patients who are more severely nearsighted, this process can take a while.

For the first four or five months, the patient will use eye drops to ensure a good result. At times, corneal haze can develop and because of this, topical steroid drops are utilized. It is unclear whether these drops will be necessary in the future, but to this point, their use has been recommended. Generally, if haze develops, it occurs at approximately four to six weeks after surgery and then tends to regress as time goes on. The best vision may not be reached for six months, or sometimes even longer in more highly myopic individuals. Once this plateau has been reached, generally the vision is stable and patients are satisfied with the results.

The early results that have been achieved at Sinai Hospital in Detroit have shown that patients who had up to -6 diopters of nearsightedness are extremely pleased with the results. The patients who have been treated for between -6 and -8 diopters of myopia have not done as well.

Laser surgery complications

What are some of the problems that can develop after Excimer Laser surgery? Corneal hazing with resultant loss of visual acuity is one concern that we will address here. In general, for the lower amounts of myopia this has not been a major problem. In addition to hazing, some people will develop glare which is reflected from the edge of the ablation. Fluctuating vision and starburst effects are not noted with the Excimer Laser. Generally, the best corrected visual acuity has been maintained although a few patients have lost one line of best corrected vision. This problem does not seem to be clinically noticeable.

In summary, I feel that Excimer Laser photorefractive keratoplasty is a safe and effective procedure, particularly for those patients who have -5 diopters or less of myopia. One advantage to it may be in its ability to more accurately correct astigmatic patients, although this again will be judged as time goes on. LASIK, as described later, is probably the best choice for myopes over -5.0 diopters.

I believe that the Excimer Laser procedure will certainly remain an option for people seeking to reduce their dependence on glasses and contacts. In the future, there will be a number of other procedures available to patients who are seeking freedom from glasses. As a surgeon, I can say that I am most excited about these endeavors, and that we are working hard to perfect all of them. For a patient who wants to be less dependent on glasses and contacts, I believe Excimer Laser photorefractive keratoplasty offers an extremely good alternative to glasses and contacts.

The remainder of this chapter was written by authors Grandon and Giffin.

Holmium Laser

While the Holmium Laser, developed by Sunrise Technology, has its greatest application in the treatment of glaucoma, there is a distinct possibility the laser could also effectively treat people with hyperopia.

The gLase™ 210 Holmium Laser System consists of a Sunrise Holmium Laser, delivery optics, slit lamp, and a table. The Sunrise System is safe, easy, and inexpensive, with the potential to surgically correct all refractive errors, although that remains a potential at this date.

The Sunrise approach makes use of the Holmium Laser to perform a special type of Laser Thermal Keratoplasty (LTK), using the principle of thermal modification of collagen, developed by Dr. Bruce Sand and known as the Sand Process. This minimally invasive procedure changes corneal shape with no pain or discomfort to the patient.

The Sunrise Corneal Shaping procedure does not cause a wound healing response. In contract to PRK, or photorefractive keratoplasty as performed by the Excimer Laser, no topical steroids are required to "manage" wound healing, and therefore there is no risk of increased intraocular pressure. In contrast to PRK, the patient's correction is believed to become stable within days after treatment.

During the Holmium Laser treatment, the patient receives a topical anesthetic and does not feel the treatment. Post-treatment, after the topical anesthetic wears off and for the first 24 hours, the patient typically experiences some foreign body sensation, but not pain. After that, the patient has normal comfort.

The Sunrise procedure causes no damage to the corneal epithelium, to Bowman's membrane, or to any other corneal microstructures. The procedure does, however, produce corneal haze in the treated spots. This haze gradually clears.

The Sunrise Corneal Shaping procedure is designed for the correction of hyperopia and astigmatism (both pre-existing and post-surgical). Correction of myopia might be a possibility in the future. How is it possible that the same laser can correct both refractive errors? Different treatment patterns and adjusted radiant exposures are used to correct different types and magnitudes of refractive error.

The Sunrise Corneal Shaping System delivers its laser energy through a slit lamp onto the patient's cornea in a predetermined treatment pattern. The patient sits upright, and his head is oriented by the standard head bar and chin rest of a slit lamp assembly. The surgeon views the patient's eye through the slit lamp and uses a laser-aiming beam to visualize the location of the laser treatment spots on the cornea.

Including patient measurements, the Sunrise procedure takes approximately 15 minutes. The actual treatment takes two seconds. The patient actively fixates on a light during this brief treatment, and the treatment pattern is centered on the pupil, with its origin placed on the patient's visual axis.

In clinical studies, patient vision has stabilized within a few months after treatment. So far, it seems to be working for lower (approximately 2D) hyperopes, but for higher degrees of hyperopia, it does not appear to be working at this time.

The Sunrise Corneal Shaping procedure is currently being investigated under an FDA-approved Investigational Device Exemption (IDE) protocol. The gLase™ 210 Laser subsystem that is part of the Sunrise Corneal Shaping System is approved for the treatment of glaucoma by the procedure of Ho: YAG laser sclerostomy.

Automated Lamellar Keratoplasty

For historical reference, Automated Lamellar Keratoplasty, also known as ALK, is another new procedure for the correction of refractive errors.

In this procedure, the surgeon cuts through 70 percent of the corneal depth to achieve correction of hyperopia; 30 percent for myopia. Then, for myopia, the surgeon makes another incision and throws away tissue to flatten the cornea. This procedure can be more dangerous than others presented in this book, because every time a surgeon cuts through the visual axis (optical zone), the result can be scarring or hazing or irregular astigmatism, which can cause permanent decrease in best corrected visual acuity. There may be increased risk involved with this procedure compared to RK.

ALK has been used to correct higher degrees of hyperopia than can be corrected with HK and the Holmium Laser, although the jury is still out on this procedure. ALK has been replaced with the new LASIK technology, which shows promise for up to -15D.

LASIK

LASIK (Laser Assisted In-situ Keratotomy) is a procedure that combines keratomileusis with the Excimer Laser for the refractive part of the surgery. It has potential for correcting degrees of myopia, hyperopia, and astigmatism, but evolving technology shows most promise for up to -15D of myopia. Chapter 15 explains LASIK in greater detail.

Laser Magic?
(This section pertains to surface laser surgery only.)
Contrary to what many people expect, lasers are not magic wands for surgeons to use to remedy any and every problem. They are not, and probably never will be, appropriate for all kinds of surgical treatments.

For the treatment of refractive errors, the Excimer Laser is still investigational in the United States and Canada. Refractive surgeons in Europe have had more extensive experience with lasers than surgeons have had here in the United States.

Cutting through the visual axis can result in irregular healing. With Excimer Laser treatment, Bowman's membrane is removed, and due to the nature of the laser's vaporization of tissue, that tissue is gone forever. We still do not know what the long-term effects of the eye are without Bowman's membrane. For this reason, and others, the FDA is still withholding approval.

In contrast to the Excimer Laser, which cuts through the visual axis, the Holmium Laser does not. The Holmium Laser treatment causes shrinkage of collagen in the periphery and a steepening in the center to decrease hyperopia. The Excimer shows possible promise for correcting astigmatism and nearsightedness, but experiments on farsighted people in Europe have not worked well.

Of course, the major difference between laser treatment and the currently accepted radial keratotomy, as well as AK, is that the traditional methods of correcting refractive error, using the diamond knife, do not cut through the visual axis, nor do they remove tissue. Because of this, the procedures are possibly safer because there is very little loss of best corrected visual acuity.

Surface Excimer and RK comparison in myopia

From Antwerp, Belgium, comes an interesting report of a case involving a patient of Dr. Luc Haverbeke. The patient specifically requested Excimer Laser treatment for his moderate degree of myopia. Because the patient had mild astigmatism in his left eye, Haverbeke persuaded him to have PRK (Excimer Laser treatment) only in the right eye and to undergo radial keratotomy in the left eye.

The patient underwent RK surgery on March 10, 1992. Using the Russian technique, Haverbeke made four incisions. On March 14, 1992, the patient underwent PRK (Excimer) on the right eye.

One week after surgery, the patient had 20/15 uncorrected visual acuity in the left eye (RK), and this result remained stable throughout the following three months. The eye was never treated with steroids during the entire postoperative period.

In the right eye (Excimer), the result was quite different. The PRK resulted in a substantial overcorrection at the one-week postoperative examination. The patient's uncorrected vision was 20/200 at one week postop. The overcorrection regressed and by three months postop, his uncorrected vision was 20/15. The patient used steroids after the procedure and will continue to use them until his cornea stabilizes. The patient complains that the vision is "hazy" when compared to the other eye.

Haverbeke has performed RK procedures for a number of years, and this case is typical of his experience, to date, with PRK (Excimer). With the PRK procedure, eyes heal slowly and unpredictably. He feels that post-PRK corneas need long-term steroid treatment and frequent monitoring. In contrast, following RK, the eye stabilizes in approximately two weeks.

PRK's unpredictable stability and visual outcome

According to an article published in 1993 in *Ophthalmology Times*, the stability and visual outcome remain unpredictable with Excimer Laser treatment.

In a study by Arthur McG. Steele, M.D., of Moorfields Eye Hospital in London, England, it was found that the outcome can be unpredictable, especially in highly myopic eyes. His conclusions were based on a recent update of the outcome of 81 patients (81 eyes) with myopia ranging from -1.5D to -10D, who underwent PRK (Excimer) and who have been carefully followed for one year. At the one-year follow-up examination, 90 percent of the patients had an uncorrected visual acuity of 20/40 or better, and 55 percent saw 20/20 or better, with the outcome depending to a great extent on their preoperative myopia. That is, 100 percent of 35 patients with a pretreatment of myopia of -4 diopters had a postoperative uncorrected visual acuity of 20/40 or better, and 55 percent saw at least 20/20.

Although the postoperative visual acuity seemed to have become "more or less stable" at the three-month examination, later tests show that many eyes had still not completely stabilized at six months and one year.

The Moorfields investigators also found that 100 percent of their patients showed some degree of corneal opacification (haze), which usually began within four to six weeks after PRK, then increased up to about six to eight months. Beyond that point, it began to subside.

In some cases, the corneal haze appeared to be associated with a loss of best corrected visual acuity. That is, 30 percent of the patients showed a loss of at least one line of best corrected vision at some time during the 12-month follow-up, persisting in 20 percent at the one-year exam.

"Some ophthalmologists may feel that a loss of only one line of best corrected visual acuity is acceptable in the face of the high level of myopic correction that can be achieved with the Excimer Laser PRK," said Steele. "However, I think we should all recognize that a loss of vision is exactly that — a loss of vision."

As for complications, 20 percent of the patients in the Moorfields study experienced glare and halos, 15 percent had reduced vision in low light, and 10 percent had occasional haziness. In fact, 43 percent of the patients had at least one of those symptoms at some time during the follow-up period. Another 11 percent had episodes of raised intraocular pressure, all of which could be controlled by withdrawing postoperative topical steroids.

"Although we found that Excimer PRK can be highly effective in most patients with low myopia and in a smaller proportion of patients in the high myopia range, unpredictability is still a problem," said Steele. "In addition, there are still many other aspects about its use that we know very little about, including how outcome is affected by age, sex, and other factors. More information about the overall utility of Excimer PRK and its long-term effects is desperately needed."

Many of the problems we have discussed in this chapter seem to be relevant only to PRK (surface laser) surgery. With LASIK, using the laser under the corneal flap, many or most problems do not seem to exist. The procedure is almost painless, and myopia, astigmatism, and hyperopia corrections seem to be quite satisfactory, but not perfect.

CHAPTER FIFTEEN
LASIK
Laser Assisted In-Situ Keratomileusis

Written by Alan Spigelman, M.D.

This chapter, also written by Dr. Alan Spigelman, introduces the reader to LASIK, which stands for Laser Assisted In-Situ Keratomileusis. The procedure is the outgrowth of work of a number of different investigators over the past 40 years. Lamellar surgery originally had its beginnings in South America. Dr. José Ignacio Barraquer began this work and developed myopic keratomileusis in approximately 1949. Initially, he developed a cryolathe. This instrument removed a section of cornea, which was frozen, reshaped on a cryolathe, and then reattached with sutures to the front of the eye. This work was extended with people working on different keratomes.

Dr. Louis Ruiz developed an automated keratome that would track across the eye on a fixed suction ring. This technology was initially used to perform automated lamellar keratoplasty (ALK), during which the keratome made both a flap and a second refractive cut. It was difficult to enhance results from automated lamellar keratoplasty, and it was felt that utilizing the laser would extend this procedure.

Dr. Ioannis Pallikaris, first coined the term LASIK. He, and other investigators, including Gholam Peyman, envisioned the use of laser under a corneal cap made by a keratome. The first LASIK procedure was performed in Europe in 1992.

LASIK has been available as an off-label usage of the Excimer Laser since 1996 in this country.

Indications

The use of LASIK for refractive surgery encompasses a fairly wide spectrum of refractive errors. It has been utilized successfully for myopia between -1 and -15 diopters. Above -15 diopters, some investigators have reported good results; however, on the horizon are intraocular lens implants that are placed over the patient's own lenses. This procedure may be a more acceptable alternative for this group of very high myopes. In addition, LASIK has been used successfully for treating astigmatism and, in fact, I have utilized it for some of my corneal transplant patients following surgery. Lastly, LASIK has been found to be acceptable for hyperopia of up to approximately 4 to 5 diopters of farsightedness. This work is more recent and is still ongoing.

Advantages

The advantages of LASIK over other refractive procedures are many. Probably the most desirable aspect of LASIK is the rapidity of return of vision for the patient. It is not uncommon for patients to return the first day after surgery with driving vision or better. Most of the patients achieve extremely good vision within the first two to three days. Visual rehabilitation can be delayed if there is any epithelial irregularity resulting from the surgery.

Secondly, LASIK results in very small amounts of discomfort. Most patients have some irritation the first evening, but by the next day the majority of patients are extremely comfortable and feel back to normal. If any epithelial irregularity results, which can occur in about 5% of the patients, discomfort may be encountered for a couple of days.

A third advantage to LASIK is the reduction of need for topical medications. Surface laser requires an extended course, approximately four months, of topical steroid. Though this is tolerated extremely well, steroids have possible side effects, including elevated intraocular pressure and cataract formation. This generally is not encountered in a course of four months, but is still a reason for follow-up examinations during that period of time. Generally, LASIK patients are kept on topical drops for one to four weeks, based on their prescription. LASIK also relies less on a patient's compliance with the drop regimen than does surface laser.

The predictability of final refractive outcome with LASIK, I feel, is slightly superior to surface laser and radial keratotomy. The result is less need for enhancements. Also, because of the highly predictable results, patients are more successfully treated with bilateral surgery. Dr. George Waring has shown that bilateral surgery gives patients less time away from work and less difficulty adapting to their new refractive state.

Lastly, I feel that the risk of infection with LASIK is exceedingly low because it is done under a corneal flap. There is no large area of abrasion for bacteria to grow. The reported incidence of infection following LASIK in this country has been extremely low. In distinction to this, there have been infections reported both with surface Excimer for refractive keratoplasty and with radial keratotomy.

However, LASIK does entail the use of a keratome to make a corneal flap [*Fig. 15*-a]. This step introduces some risk to the procedure. We will touch on flap complications at the end of this chapter, but in deciding to do LASIK, it is best to choose a surgeon who feels comfortable with this technique.

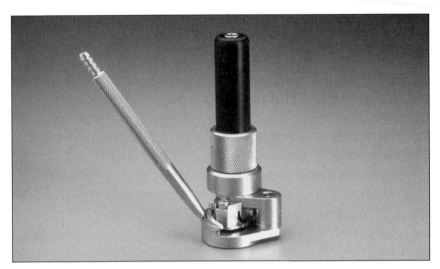

Fig. 15-a With the keratome, the surgeon makes the corneal flap.

Patient selection

Patients are selecting refractive surgery for a number of reasons, including the ability to pursue active lifestyles without the need for glasses or contact lenses, engage in professions that require less dependence on corrective lenses, avoid the headache of using contact lenses and solutions, and to enjoy the cosmetic appearance of being free of glasses.

Refractive procedures are for patients with essentially healthy eyes. A patient undergoing any refractive procedure will need to be examined carefully by the surgeon to rule out any possible eye diseases, including keratoconus (an abnormal shape of the cornea). It is also, in general, not for patients who have significant systemic disease. In particular, all immune diseases, such as rheumatoid arthritis and systemic lupus erythematosus, are not compatible with good results with any of the refractive procedures. It is important to make your surgeon aware of any diseases that you have so that these can be considered prior to refractive surgery.

Patient preparation

Once the patient has decided to pursue LASIK surgery, the surgeon will discuss what is to be expected during surgery. It is important to know that vision is generally dimmed as the keratome passes across the eye, because of the suction ring increasing the intraocular pressure. This usually lasts for 15 to 30 seconds. Once the keratome passes completely, it is important for the patient to fixate on the fixation light. The surgeon will encourage the patient to continue looking toward that area even when the light seems to blur out.

The surgeon has the ability to start and stop the treatment at any time, so if the patient fixation is lost, the laser treatment is not decentered. It is important for the patient to understand that the surgeon is focusing and centering the laser so that he does not feel that any small movement of the eye will cause a poor result. In general, patients are able to fixate the light quite easily, and this does not seem to be a problem for patients.

When the patient arrives at the laser center, he is generally given a small amount of sedation with oral Valium, and then undergoes a surgical preparation of the eyelids using a surgical scrub. It is important not to wear makeup or perfumes on the day of surgery. They can impact on the mirrors of the laser and also create more debris that could potentially get underneath the corneal flap.

The patient is then brought into the surgical suite where he is placed under the laser and put into position. If the VISX Star Laser is being utilized, the laser at that point will undergo a self-calibration cycle allowing the patient to hear what the laser sounds like.

Once this is completed, a lid speculum is placed onto the eye. The speculum holds the eyelid open and prevents the patient from blinking during the procedure. This is a very important point, and it reassures the patient that he cannot cause a problem by blinking. The speculum is usually the most uncomfortable aspect of the surgery, particularly for patients who have small orbits, or eyes, in lay terms.

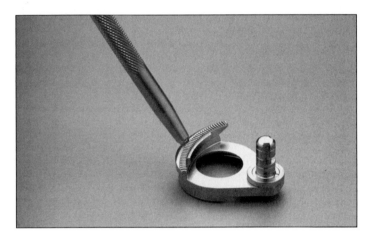

Fig. 15-b The suction ring prevents the eye from moving.

Next, the suction ring is applied to the eye and turned on. *Fig. 15-b.* This is when the vision may blur out. The keratome is placed onto the track of the suction ring and passed across the eye. Generally, this is about a 15- to 30-second procedure, in total.

Once the flap has been accomplished, the suction ring is entirely removed from the eye. The patient has the flap pulled back and is instructed to look at the blinking red light. Typically, the treatment time lasts between 30 and 80 seconds, depending on the patient's prescription. *Fig. 15-c.*

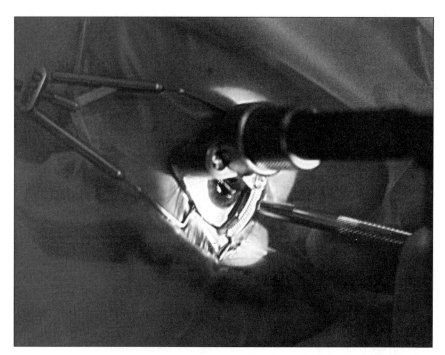

Fig. 15-c The keratome is attached to the suction ring for LASIK surgery.

When the laser treatment has been entirely accomplished, the flap is put back into place and allowed to dry for approximately three minutes. This done, the second eye can undergo LASIK if this has been planned in advance.

The patient is then taken out of the laser suite and returned to the examining room. Approximately five minutes later, the patient is examined with the slit lamp to ensure that the flap placement is good. If there is any problem with the flap position at that time, the patient can be returned to the surgical suite and have it replaced. This is uncommon, but it adds a safeguard for the patient.

Postoperatively, the patient can expect mild to moderate discomfort for the first evening. Usually upon awakening the next day, the patient will notice improved vision and absence of pain. It is not uncommon for patients to drive to the doctor's office the next day, nor is it uncommon for patients to return to work the next day. However, if one day can be taken after surgery for recuperation, it would be advisable.

Results

I believe that, in general, 95% of the patients who are considered to be good candidates for LASIK will achieve 20/40 or better vision. Just as a generality, about 50 to 70 percent will achieve 20/25 vision or better, and probably 80 to 90% will achieve 20/30 or better. I believe that most patients are extremely satisfied with their vision when it reaches 20/30 or better. Some patients are satisfied with 20/40 vision, although others may feel this is not sufficient vision even though it meets driver's license qualifications. If the patient and physician feel that vision can be improved, a second procedure can be undertaken, usually two to six months later.

The second procedure, or enhancement, can be performed either by recutting a new flap using the keratome or by picking up the old flap and adding additional laser treatment. The decision of just how to approach this can be discussed with the surgeon. There are pros and cons to both of these approaches, although, in general, if someone has had surgery six months or more prior, it is probably best to cut a new flap.

Complications

The vast majority of patients who undergo LASIK surgery will encounter no difficulties with the procedure at all. However, no procedure is done without risk.

Probably the biggest risk to any refractive procedure is that patients do not achieve 20/20 vision without glasses. When someone is considering this surgery, it is best to understand that one may not achieve exactly the vision that had been attained with glasses or contacts in the past.

The surgery will give patients independence from contact lenses and glasses; and the majority of time, they will need no glasses to improve vision. This procedure also does not remove the need for reading glasses when patients reach their 40s and 50s. Occasionally, patients will note that if they have a slight amount of residual nearsightedness, they can read well, function in the office quite well, drive during the day, but find that they need driving glasses in the evening. This may be a suitable alternative for a number of patients who have desk-type jobs during the day.

Another inter-operative problem is what we term a *free cap*. Instead of having a hinge at the edge of the LASIK resection, the cap is unhinged from the cornea and can be totally removed. In fact, this is not really a complication. It was the manner in which early automated lamellar keratoplasties were carried out. It takes a little more time to reposition the flap after surgery, and generally the surgeon will let it dry on the eye for a longer period of time. Usually it can be handled well, and I do not believe that this is a significant issue.

One issue that can be significant is *corneal epithelial defects*. The patients who have epithelial defects may be fit with a bandage contact lens at the end of the procedure and need to be watched for healing. The concern is that epithelium can grow underneath the flap that can cause irregularities of the vision and significant problems. If epithelium is under the flap, frequently it can just be observed. However, if it is growing, the surgeon will probably recommend to go back underneath the flap and scrape it out. Generally, this can be accomplished successfully but it can lead to some degradation of vision.

During the procedure, if the keratome stops prior to completing the pass, a short flap or irregular flap can be encountered. As long as the keratome does not stop within the visual axis, this is usually not a problem. However, the completion of surgery probably cannot occur for approximately two to three months. It is best, if the flap is not perfect, to just replace it at the time of surgery. It will heal back without any scarring, and then the surgeon can go back to accomplish a better flap at a later time after the cornea has healed.

One of the most serious complications during surgery can be loss of suction. If the suction breaks during the procedure, the keratome can cut an unusual shaped flap or perforate the flap centrally. This will generally result in irregularity in the center of the vision and possibly induce epithelial ingrowth. This can be very difficult to fix. If it does occur, it is best for the surgeon to replace the flap as perfectly as possible and let it heal. A superficial keratectomy or a photorefractive keratoplasty can be carried out later, removing any haze that might have developed. Generally, patients who have this happen may have a degradation of their vision, but, hopefully, if care is taken in repositioning the flap, the loss of vision can be kept to a very minimal amount. This complication is extremely rare, but it is possible.

Infection, as mentioned earlier, is very uncommon with LASIK, and may occur once in 5,000 procedures, based on international experience. A sterile technique is used for cleaning surgical instruments, and patients are given antibiotics to use after surgery.

Lastly, some patients may have some fluctuation in their vision. This is much less common than it is with radial keratotomy; however, it can still be noted for the first few months. Additionally, night glare can be a factor for some patients. It is particularly true for patients who have high degrees of nearsightedness or who have pupils that dilate very widely in a dark environment. Hopefully, if a patient has a widely dilated pupil in the dark, it will be noted by the surgeon prior to surgery; at least, this can be discussed. It has been uncommon in my experience for patients to complain of fluctuating vision or night glare after a three- to six-month period of time following surgery.

Conclusion

LASIK has greatly enhanced our armamentarium for treating nearsightedness, astigmatism and, down the road, farsightedness. Acceptance by patients has been extremely high. I believe that, with proper patient preparation and understanding, the vast majority of patients will be extremely happy with their outcome. Still, LASIK is a surgical procedure and it needs to be undertaken by any prospective patient with care. Based on my experiences and on others around the country, the vast majority of patients have obtained extremely gratifying results.

My commitment to LASIK is complete. I underwent the procedure in June of 1998. My motivation was twofold. First was my desire to no longer wear glasses. My preoperative vision was -5.50 diopters of myopia. In the second place, I felt uncomfortable recommending LASIK to patients without having undergone it myself.

As with any other patient, I was nervous about having this surgery done. I understood the risk involved, but I also knew that out of more than 500 patients on whom I had performed surgery, no one had lost significant vision. The majority of my patients, in fact, were thrilled. I had operated on my sister in April of 1998, and her encouragement prompted me to schedule my own surgery.

The surgery day was surprisingly uneventful. I was excited and anticipated a good result. The surgery itself was almost entirely painless and lasted less than 15 minutes. Throughout the procedure, I kept thinking about how I would be doing it. I also realized that my fixation on the red light was crucial. I was entirely focused on this light during the actual laser treatment, which lasted about 25 seconds in each eye.

Immediately following surgery my vision was cloudy, but I could see where I was going. I kept my eyes shut for two hours. Then I had dinner and watched TV. When I awoke the next day, I could see that my distance vision was great. My near vision was more blurred. When I saw the doctor the next day, my vision was 20/30 in my right eye and 20/50 in my left eye. Both eyes were slightly farsighted. This has improved over the first month, and now my vision is 20/20 in my right eye and 20/25 in my left eye.

Overall, I am ecstatic! The quality of my vision in many respects is better than it was with glasses. I find that my vision continues to improve. Even though my surgery was only two months ago, it is hard for me to believe I ever wore glasses.

CHAPTER SIXTEEN
Hyperopic LASIK

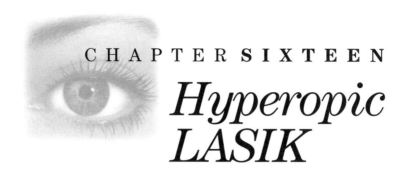

LASIK for hyperopia (farsightedness)

In the original keratomileusis procedure for myopia, Dr. José Ignacio Barraquer removed a slice of the cornea with a microkeratome, froze it, lathe cut it, and sutured it back onto the cornea.

For hyperopia, seven or eight years ago, he made a deep cut through the center of the cornea that caused a bulging (weakening) in front of the eye, due to pressure, and therefore corrected hyperopia. The problem was that it was not predictable. If the cut was too deep, there was a possibility that the patient would need corneal transplants. Although most people did well, there was a higher risk of complication. Now, hyperopic LASIK is being done on an investigational basis in the United States.

Dr. Klaus Ditzen, Dr. Helda Huschka, and Stefan Pieger, Msc, studied forty-three hyperopic patients (19 men, 24 women) between 18 and 40 years (mean age, 37) who had had LASIK for hyperopia during a period of one year (September 1994 to September 1995).

After surgery, the patients were examined daily for one week, then at intervals of one, two, three, six, and 12 months.

Surgical Procedure

Topical anesthetic is administered over one hour before surgery, and a lid speculum is used to keep the eyelids open. The optical center of the cornea is marked with a special marker. The suction ring is placed on the eye, and vacuum is created to hold the fixation ring onto the globe and create a rigid corneal surface in order to get a perfect cut.

The diameter of the corneal flap is 8.5mm (with the newer Hansatome, it is about 9.3mm), and the thickness of the flap is set. After measuring the intraocular pressure and adjusting the flap diameter, the microkeratome is placed into the tract of the suction ring.

A corneal flap with a small hinge is created, and the flap is opened. The flap is lifted. The patient looks at the fixation light in the laser, then the photoablation is carried out. The center of the cornea is steepened by removing peripheral tissue from the sides.

After the laser procedure, the flap is repositioned, and the edge dried with sponges. Immediately after the procedure, three drops each of homoatropine, antibiotics, and a nonsteroidal anti-inflammatory are administered.

For the first four postoperative days, antibiotics are given three times a day. Fluorometolone (steroid) eyedrops three times a day are maintained for four weeks, with the dosage eventually reduced to one drop a day weekly.

Efficacy

Generally, best corrected visual acuity, in the patients studied, had stabilized after one week. Ninety-five percent of the corrected hyperopic eyes with a preoperative refraction of up to +4D achieved an uncorrected visual acuity of 20/40 or better; 90% achieved this acuity in the +4.25D to +8D group. There was 5% loss of one Snellen line caused by epithelial ingrowth.

Complications

In this particular study, epithelial ingrowth was the most common complication, with 15%. Mostly, it was observed in higher hyperopes and where they had problems with the suction ring or with the microkeratome blade. A possible reason could also be the cleaning technique, as the surgeons did not clean the flap before repositioning. Flap dislocations and fold flaps seemed to be caused by intraoperative complications with the suction, the blade, or the stopper device. [Again, with the newest Hansatome Keratome technology, some of these complications will probably be eliminated.]

Haze was seen in only one patient, and that was eventually reduced significantly. In only three cases were scars observed, due to the laser beam touching the inside of the hinge.

There were two cases of decentration, occurring in eyes with high hyperopia (+7 and +9, with a corneal diameter of 9.5mm). In each case, the suction ring could not be fixed well enough to the globe during the operation because the diameter of the suction ring was too large.

Conclusions

The surgeons in this study found that LASIK for hyperopia has a better predictability, stability, efficacy, and safety than surface PRK, especially in higher hyperopic eyes with more than +3D of hyperopia.

Although hyoperopic LASIK is still in the early stages of development, with the latest keratome technology, we are confident that LASIK will become a valuable alternative for the correction of hyperopia, and for the correction of myopic LASIK procedures that resulted in hyperopia. Also, LASIK will be used for the correction of overcorrected radial keratotomy procedures.

With the new Hansatome Keratome technology, we expect some of the complications reviewed in this chapter, such as epithelial downgrowth, to be greatly minimized if not completely eliminated. For hyperopic LASIK, the surgeon needs to make a bigger flap, so when doing hyperopia correction with the Hansatome Keratome, we expect the results to be improved over the results noted in this study.

The FDA has recently approved the Excimer Laser for treatment of up to +6 diopters of hyperopia.

CHAPTER SEVENTEEN
The Refractive Intra-ocular Lens

Written by Henry Hirschman, M.D.

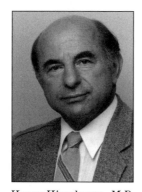

Henry Hirschman, M.D.

The author, Henry Hirschman, M.D., was the first in the world to combine phacoemulsification with IOL implantation in 1969, and he performed the first modern lens implant in the West in 1967. [There were some physicians, including Dr. Frank Markey, who took the technique from Europe in the early 1950s. Those fell out of favor because the technology was not advanced.] Dr. Hirschman has since lectured on IOLs all over the world, has invented numerous IOL surgical instruments, and has authored many books and articles for prestigious ophthalmology journals.

Glasses and contact lenses have been an enormous boon and have helped millions of people enjoy fuller lives, but they have not been an unmixed blessing. They do nothing to correct the basic refractive error. Glasses allow people with mild to moderate errors to function fairly well, but the *very* nearsighted or farsighted person is totally dependent on glasses or contacts, and that is, to say the least, undesirable.

The case of cataract patients is particularly poignant. A cataract is a clouding of the natural lens of the eye. For centuries, the only treatment has been, and remains, surgical removal. This procedure, however, left the patient without the optical benefit of the natural lens, and therefore left them out of focus. Cataract surgery made people very farsighted. For many years, thick, strong "Coke bottle" lenses were the only way that these people could see. (Relatively few were able to handle contact lenses for any length of time.)

In 1949, one of the truly rare "breakthroughs" in medicine occurred. Harold Ridley fashioned an artificial lens that he implanted in the eye of a cataract patient. While far from perfect, the procedure worked well enough to encourage further refinement, and today virtually all cataract patients have the benefit of an intra-ocular lens that has been customized to the exact power and size for each patient. "Coke bottle" glasses are no longer seen. *Lens replacement* has been added to *lens removal*, and many millions of cataract patients have been given a new lease on life. Many are seeing better *without* glasses than they ever saw *with* them. Improvements in design and manufacture now approach perfection, and our experience showing their safety is measured in decades.

What about those who do not have cataracts, but who are nevertheless dependent on glasses? There are certainly a lot of people in this world who are so farsighted or nearsighted that they must wear glasses from the first thing in the morning until bedtime.

It has been determined that most of these people can have the benefit of modern intra-ocular lens (IOL) technology and microsurgery. Instead of designing a lens to *replace* the natural lens of the eye, lenses have been designed, and used, to *supplement* and actually correct severe refractive errors; i.e., the very nearsighted and the very farsighted.

Since the natural lens is left undisturbed, the operation is much simpler than the cataract procedure. The entire operation consists of making a small (1/4 inch) incision at the edge of the cornea and placing the appropriate tiny lens in the space between the iris and the cornea (the anterior chamber). One or two stitches are used to close the incision.

More than a million lenses of similar design have been used in cataract surgery for more than 20 years, as a replacement for the cloudy natural lens. We have had a great deal of experience with them. Today's lenses have a flawless finish, extreme flexibility, and excellent optics.

Almost all of the available refractive surgery procedures achieve their result by flattening the corneal curvature so that the total refractive power of the eye is reduced. This corrects myopia. The laser procedures do this by thinning the central part of the cornea. The more myopia that needs correction, the more corneal tissue must be removed. Attempts at correcting high myopia suffers from a drop in the accuracy and the stability of the correction. For this reason, the best laser results are in the low to moderate range of myopia. The laser has not been very effective in the treatment of farsightedness.

Those who favor the use of the phakic IOL can cite the following advantages:
- The refractive IOL is equally effective in the treatment of nearsightedness (myopia) and farsightedness (hyperopia). It is useful in the hyperopic range from +2.0 to +10.0 diopters and in myopia from -5.00 diopters to -20.00.
- There is no thinning of the cornea.
- The accuracy and predictability is superior to all other modalities.
- The recovery time is short: One day.

- The results are stable.
- The procedure is entirely reversible, should that ever become necessary.
- The lens material has been used in the eye for 50 years.
- The basic lens design has been in use for more than 20 years.
- The quality of vision is unsurpassed, since there is no incision in the visual axis.
- Previously seen complications of ovalization of the pupil and progressive endothelial cell loss have been eliminated.

This approach has been used all over the world for the past decade, and will be available in the United States soon.

[As of this writing in mid-1998, the Phakic IOL procedure has not been approved by the Food & Drug Administration. The procedures are being performed in core studies throughout the United States, but in many parts of the world they are being done on a routine basis with excellent results.]

CHAPTER **EIGHTEEN**

Lens Extraction and Intra-ocular Lens Implant

Written by **Dennis L. Williams, M.D.**
St. Luke's Cataract & Laser Institute
Tarpon Springs, Florida

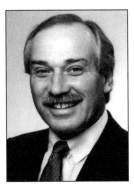

Dennis L. Williams, M.D.

The author, Dennis L. Williams, M.D., selected by his peers as one of the best doctors in the Southeast United States, has a 10-year follow-up on patients whose myopia was -25.00 diopters or greater of myopia or 4 diopters or greater of hyperopia. Dr. Williams has performed more secondary intraocular implants than any other eye surgeon in the United States.

Also known as *clear lensectomy*, the lens extraction and intraocular lens implant procedure takes off where radial keratotomy and laser surgery (PRK/LASIK) — and their effectiveness for patients with high amounts of myopia and hyperopia — ends.

The natural lens is removed, as with cataract surgery, and a plastic intraocular prescription lens is inserted. The artificial lens has a set focus and cannot zoom in and out to change focus. Recently, however, artificial lenses of variable focus capabilities have been inserted in cataract patients with success.

With a set focus intra-ocular lens, the patient must wear reading glasses or have each eye implanted with a distance correction for the dominant eye, and a near correction for the non-dominant eye. This "one for near and one for far" procedure has successfully been performed with contact lenses, radial keratotomy, laser surgery, and cataract surgery, and is known as *monovision*. Monovision allows patients to see well enough to pass a driver's test without spectacles and still be able to read.

The clear lens extraction has been performed by a limited number of surgeons in the United States and the world. The procedure has appealed to cataract surgeons with extensive experience in calculating accurate lens power and performing small-incision surgery with minimal induced astigmatism or correcting preexisting astigmatism with astigmatic keratotomy incisions. As an added bonus, the patient will never require a cataract operation in the future.

The ideal candidate for clear lensectomy is a patient whose eyeglass lens prescription registers in double digits, i.e., -10 diopters or greater of myopia or 4 diopters or greater of hyperopia. The clear lens extraction carries the same risk of complications as cataract surgery that is performed successfully over a million times a year in the United States.

In comparing patients who have had laser surgery in one eye and clear lensectomy in the second eye, patients prefer the clarity of the intraocular lens eye over the lasered eye, even though both eyes were seeing 20/20 based on the eye chart.

A new variation of this technique is being investigated by the FDA in the United States. In that procedure, a soft intraocular lens is placed between the cornea and the natural crystalline lens of the eye, which is, essentially, a contact lens for the natural lens of the eye. One of the complications of this procedure is the development of cataracts and the development of pupillary block glaucoma.

In summary, the clear lens extraction is a safe and effective procedure for patients with large amounts of myopia and hyperopia that cannot be corrected with RK or laser surgery.

CHAPTER NINETEEN
Computers in Refractive Surgery

Written by **Gary M. Grandon, Ph.D.**

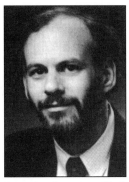

Gary M. Grandon, Ph.D.

The author of this chapter is Dr. Stanley C. Grandon's brother, Gary M. Grandon, Ph.D., Associate Vice Chancellor for Computing and Imaging Systems at the University of North Carolina (Greensboro). They combined their areas of expertise to create predictability software that has enabled Dr. Grandon to achieve some of the best RK results in the world. We present it primarily for historical interest; however, we still use the software on RKs we perform today, and other ophthalmologists around the world also continue to use it.)

Computers in radial keratotomy surgery

Today, computers are used in nearly every aspect of human life. In surgical ophthalmology, they are only now beginning to reveal their potential.

Computers are invaluable for two important aspects of RK surgery:

- statistical analysis and medical record maintenance, and

- production of "expert systems," computer programs with which the surgeon consults to determine precisely what surgical parameters he will use for an individual surgery.

This chapter is divided into two general parts. The first discusses how the computer has allowed RK surgeons to analyze the massive amount of data which is collected on RK patients. This second part discusses the development of KeraStat™, a powerful RK expert system.

From this point on, we will focus on the findings and procedures used by Dr. Stanley C. Grandon and Gary M. Grandon, Ph.D., who took on the continued maintenance and analysis of Grandon's surgical data after the ARK Study Group was disbanded.

Out of fairness to other ophthalmic surgeons who perform radial keratotomy, we would like to mention that excellent software programs have also been developed by Bores, Dietz, Kremer, and Arrowsmith, as well as Drs. Spencer Thornton and Frank Grady.

Statistical analysis and medical records

Patient data collection

At the time of this writing, data has been amassed on more than 10,000 RK surgeries performed by Dr. Stanley Grandon.

In addition to measurements made of the patient's eyes during his initial visit, additional data are collected during surgery on the size and shape of the clear zone used, depth of the incisions, types of incisions, and knife used. All patient data are recorded on special intake forms.

After surgery, patient follow-up visits are carefully recorded, noting such data as refraction, corneal curvature, visual acuity, intraocular pressure, postoperative symptoms of discomfort, medication, and other subjective findings.

These forms are then sent to Gary Grandon, where they are entered into a microcomputer database system to be verified and rechecked for accuracy. The amount of data now on hand is too massive for microcomputer analysis. Once satisfied with their accuracy, the data (now in computer form) are sent by electronic communication to the mainframe host computer systems at the University of North Carolina at Greensboro. There they are added to the entire RK database, from which selected groups of patients are used for specific research studies.

Of course, the major concern is long term follow-up on RK patients. Using standard statistical software systems and specialized programming techniques, a number of reports and studies have been produced by Drs. Grandon. They have also utilized these data to produce a powerful RK expert system.

RK results by Dr. Stanley Grandon

As Mark Twain said, "There are lies, damn lies, and statistics." The key to understanding statistical data rests in knowing what specific patients are being compared to which others.

A word about these cases. "We are quite careful in making claims (our lawyers keep us that way)," said Gary Grandon. "What we are reporting here are results after the first RK surgery. Many patients, who do not achieve optimal results after a single surgery, can and do have another RK procedure.

After the second surgery, their vision is almost always better. We report these more conservative 'first surgery' findings here so as not to confuse the readers of other studies and to let them know just what they are looking at."

Unfortunately, most readers do not think in terms of *diopters of spherical equivalent* (whatever that is!). They think in terms of the more familiar 20/20, 20/40 type of measurement. This type of measurement is known as visual acuity or 'how well you can see when you try.' How we are using measurements of visual acuity without corrective lenses (without glasses or contacts).

Here then are the Eye Surgery Institute's findings in terms of how well patients can actually see after surgery. One problem with visual acuity, though, is that many patients are worse than 20/400 without correction before surgery. So the diopter method to assess preoperative myopia will have to be used.

Here are some rules of thumb. Patients with less than -3 diopters of myopia may not need to wear corrective lenses all of the time. Patients worse than -6 diopters are considered high myopes who cannot function at all without thick corrective lenses. *Fig. 19-a.*

Postoperative Visual Acuity RK Patients Three Months or More After Surgery Eight Incision Cases by Preop S.E.

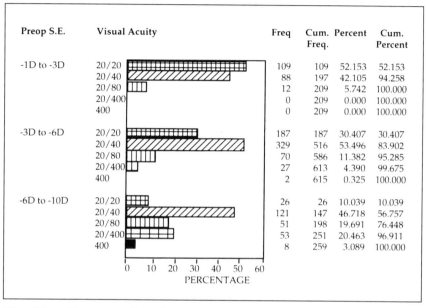

Fig. 19-a Postoperative visual acuity for RK patients by degree of preoperative myopia

If you are nearsighted, you can use *Fig. 19-a* to judge the visual outcome of RK for yourself. It is divided into the three groups of patients mentioned above. If you qualify for RK surgery, you can use your corrective lens prescription to determine where you enter the chart. Take the first number (the sphere — if it's not a negative number, consult your eye doctor before using this chart) and add one-half the second number (the cylinder) to it. This yields what is called the *spherical equivalent* or your myopia without astigmatism. If this number is between -1 and -3, about 50% of patients with similar myopia have achieved 20/20 or better vision after RK. Likewise, 94% have achieved 20/40 or better vision after RK. Few patients with 20/40 or better vision require glasses for most activities.

Likewise, if you have high myopia (-6 to -10 diopters). Fifty-six percent of other RK patients in a similar situation have achieved 20/40 or better vision.

Some researchers have recently reported that vision after RK surgery may not be stable for all patients. This means that the refraction of some patients may change in time.[1] The Grandons have also investigated changes in vision of their RK patients.[2]

"We found that 89% of eight-incision, non-astigmatic RK patients had no significant shift in their refractions from three months after surgery to three years after surgery," said Grandon. "We also found, in a control group of patients, that only 76.9% of these patients, who had not undergone RK surgery but who could have been candidates for the surgery, had stable vision for that three-year period. And after statistically controlling for preoperative differences in myopia other measures (mentioned previously), we found no significant differences in vision from three months to one year, two years, or three years."

Physicians at the Eye Surgery Institute believe that changes in vision occur as people mature, that those shifts reported, on average, are small (about .5 diopters). And that by carefully controlling which patients are compared to each other, these shifts are not a matter of RK surgery but simply a matter of patient maturity. For the majority of his RK patients, Grandon has found no important changes in long-term vision.

Expert systems — using the computer to make RK better

Prediction Equations

A second way in which computers are used in RK surgery is for the development of expert systems to help the surgeon determine the best parameters for an individual's surgery. These systems are developed using a combination of techniques, including data analysis, statistical modeling, and artificial intelligence computer programming techniques.

Statisticians have developed very sophisticated mathematical techniques for predicting the outcomes of various events. Unfortunately, they are not always perfect. Individuals sometimes react differently to various treatments. For example, taking aspirin does not always cure a headache; flu shots do not always prevent the flu; and glasses do not always correct one's vision. So, too, with RK surgery. Individuals react somewhat differently from one another. The important thing to remember is that statistical techniques cannot always indicate how well they are able to predict an outcome. And when presented properly to the physician, adjustments in surgical parameters can be made to achieve the best possible results.

As you may be aware, a poor outcome for a patient who has been nearsighted all his life is to be made significantly farsighted. When you are nearsighted, distant objects may be blurry, but you can still see things up close. When you are farsighted, you lose your ability to see things which are close.[3] Most patients would prefer to remain a little nearsighted than be significantly farsighted. It is very important to consider carefully the chances of overcorrection in RK surgery. So, special attention has been paid to statistical techniques which provide information on the confidence in the predictions that are being made.

Predicting RK results

Before computers were used to examine the predictability of RK outcomes, tables of numbers (called *nomograms*) or special 'rule of thumb' formulae [4] were used to determine parameters of surgery. Unfortunately, none of these techniques can provide information on the confidence of a predicted outcome for a specific patient.

The Grandons and others have turned then to a technique called *Multiple Regression Analysis*, which is able to examine how well a particular combination of predictors fits known outcomes of RK surgery (i.e., the change in myopia after RK surgery). They have taken the battery of preoperative data described earlier and determined which predictors best indicate the correction in myopia after RK surgery. After studying how these prediction equations behave, they were able to confirm several theoretical problems. The first of these is called *regression toward the mean*.

Regression toward the mean is an effect that numerically forced 'predicted results' (from regression equations) to be more closely bunched around the 'average' result of the calibration cases than they should be. That is, the original cases are more different from one another than the predicted outcomes from the equations would have you believe. This is particularly true for cases of low and high myopia. Ignoring this fact can cause overcorrection.

To better control for this effect, the Grandons have generated four separate regression formulae, one for each range of preoperative myopia and a fourth overall equation. This minimizes the systematic statistical effects of regression toward the mean. [5]

Another important feature of regression techniques is the fact that for a given patient, the degree of confidence a physician has in a predicted outcome depends on how much that patient is like the average patient in the calibration group (the patients on whom the equations are calculated). They use a statistical measure called the *standard error of prediction*, which includes distance measures from the composite of preoperative measures on the current patient, and the average patient in the calibration group. Again, this provides the physician with a very useful confidence index.

Kera-Stat — an expert RK computer system

In order to make the Eye Surgery Institute's statistical findings translate back into surgical practice, the Grandons have developed a microcomputer program which can be used in a physician's office. Although the database management and statistical analyses require greater computer power than is readily available in a physician's office, the regression equations and specific RK patient preoperative data can be calculated and maintained on a typical business microcomputer.

Kera-Stat was developed to provide the RK surgeon with all the information and clinical experience gained from more than 5,000 cases of RK surgery and several years of statistical analysis of outcomes. The physician enters patient preoperative data. *Fig. 19-b.*

Kera-Stat Modify Patient Data

Enter Record Number of 9999 for New Case

Record Number: 1
Case Number: 0010-1-0 <-

Patient Name: Jane Smith
Age: 39
I.O.P. 19.5
Axial Length: 24
Average Keratotomy: 44.2
Sex (1=Male/2=Female): 2

Pre Op Sphere: -5
Pre Op Cylinder (+): 3
Pre Op Axis: 45

Post Op Sphere: 0
Post Op Cylinder (+): 0
Post Op Axis: 0

'Return' to Change Value, 'End' to Save,
'ESC' to Quit, '<-' or '->'

Fig. 19-b Kera-Stat patient data screen with sample patient information

Then he selects the appropriate statistical model (or the overall model for all ranges of myopia). *Fig. 19-c.*

CHAPTER NINETEEN COMPUTERS IN REFRACTIVE SURGERY

Current Patient:
    Record Number: 1
    Case Number: 0010-1-0
    Patient Name: Jane Smith

Enter the Number of the Option You Wish to Use and Press 'RETURN'. . .

1. MODEL 1 Pre-operative up to -11
2. MODEL 2 Pre-operative Less Than or Equal -3
3. MODEL 3 Pre-operative -3 to -6
4. MODEL 4 Pre-operative Greater Than or Equal -6
5. Modify/Add Patient Data
6. Find Patient by Case Number
7. Set Physician Depth Factor. . .Currently 0 Percent
8. Exit System. . .

Enter Number of Selection=>?

Fig. 19-c Kera-Stat main option menu indicating program features

The system then calculates predicted outcomes for various types of RK surgery for that particular patient. *Fig. 19-d.*

Raw Corrections in Diopters - Model 3.
Spherical 8-Incisions -3 to -6D

Number 1 Case: 0010-1-0 Name: Jane Smith Age=39 Phys. Dpth Factor=0%
Axial Length=24   I.O.P.= 19.5 Ave. Kera= 44.2   Sex=F

Clear Zone Sizes	85%	Expected Incision Depth 90%	95%	Average
3	3.341	3.787	4.233	4.160
Confidence	0.863	0.852	0.848	
3.5	2.834	3.280	3.726	3.653
Confidence	0.858	0.847	0.843	
4	2.326	2.773	3.219	3.146
Confidence	0.857	0.845	0.841	
4.5	1.819	2.266	2.712	2.639
Confidence	0.859	0.847	0.843	
5	1.312	1.758	2.205	
Confidence	0.864	0.851	0.847	
5.5	0.805	1.251	1.698	1.624
Confidence	0.872	0.859	0.855	

Note: 68% of Cases fall within the Confidence Interval
         95% fall within 2 times the Confidence Interval
Enter (Y/N) for Surgical Recommendations=>?

Fig. 19-d Kera-Stat table of expected changes in spherical equivalent for sample patient including confidence intervals

From the information in *Fig. 19-d*, an experienced RK surgeon could determine parameters for a specific surgery, but the Grandons have not stopped here.

Computers have the ability to examine information and, according to pre-programmed rules, they are able to make decisions among various alternatives. When computer programs are able to make these decisions 'intelligently,' they are sometimes called *artificially intelligent systems*. When they behave as if they were a human expert in a particular content area, they are termed expert systems. Kera-Stat is an expert RK system. The Grandons have, over the past few years, added to this simple table of numbers [*Fig. 19-d*] specific recommendations for surgery. *Fig. 19-e.*

Surgical recommendations using the Grandon technique

```
For Record Number: 1
        Case Number:      0010-1-0
        Patient Name:     Jane Smith

        Initial Refraction:    -5      3      45

        Astigmatic Correction: .    4 Flags at 7mm.

        Incision Depth:       95%

        Number of Incisions:  Eight

        Elliptical Clear Zone: Major Axis= 5.25   Minor Axis= 4.75

        Total Expected Correction:    4.125054

        Do You Wish to See a Graphic Representation (Y/N)=>?
```

Fig. 19-e Kera-Stat expert surgical recommendations for sample patient

These recommendations vary for each specific patient according to the collective experience of all the cases performed by Grandon. In a sense, Kera-Stat is 'Grandons in a box.' In order to make sure of the recommendations in the operating room, Kera-Stat shows a picture of the surgical procedure which can be printed onto paper. *Fig. 19-f.*

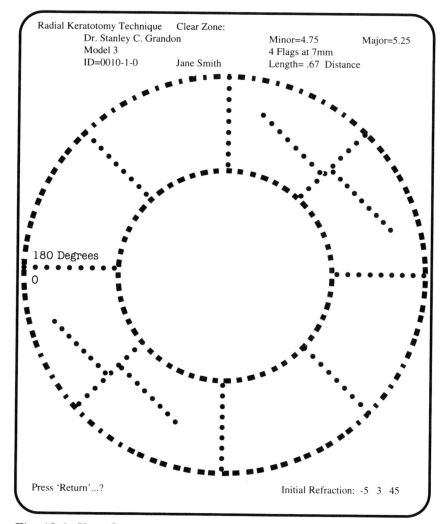

Fig. 19-f Kera-Stat expert surgical recommendation for sample patient — graphic display of surgery. The radial lines indicate the location of the incisions. The four cross lines indicate the location of the flag incisions designed to correct astigmatism.

Conclusion

The computer has made its presence known to the RK surgeon. It has proved to be an invaluable tool with which to conduct research, as well as a trustworthy colleague. It will always continue to be used in these and even more impressive ways.

Footnotes

[1] Reports were made of findings from Dietz's early RK surgeries: Dietz MR, Sanders DR, Raana MG, <u>Progressive Hyperopia in Radial Keratotomy</u>. Ophthalmology, Vol. 93, Number 10, October, 1986.

[2] They presented their findings: Grandon SC, Grandon GM, <u>Comparison of Refractive Stability in RK Patients and Control Group</u>. Presentation to the Kerato-Refractive Surgery Society, 1986.

[3] This is quite different from presbyopia, which requires bifocal lenses. Presbyopia is associated with the eye's losing its ability to accommodate (or change shape) as one gets older. This causes the closest point at which you can focus to get further from your eye. Although sometimes confused with nearsightedness, it is quite different.

[4] Fyodorov's formula is one of these. An exception to the rule of thumb formula, which has been used successfully, is the more complicated model developed by Schachar and Drs. Truman D. Black and Tseng Huang in their book <u>Understanding Radial Keratotomy</u> (LAL Publishing, Denison, TX, 1981). This excellent model is still the best theoretical basis for experimentation today.

[5] The Grandons have also found the influence of different groups of patient myopia. See Grandon GM, Grandon SC. <u>Causal Analysis of RK Outcomes, A Computer Analysis.</u> Proceedings of the Refractive Surgery Society's Annual Meeting, 1986.

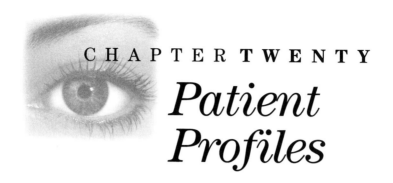

CHAPTER TWENTY
Patient Profiles

Many thousands of patients have achieved excellent vision as a result of refractive surgery. A few of Dr. Grandon's former patients expressed an interest in publicly discussing their pre-operative conditions, as well as their experience undergoing surgery and, particularly, their life with new vision. Here are their stories.

DALE, a police officer

> Right eye before surgery - Count fingers
> Right eye after surgery - 20/15
>
> Left eye before surgery - Count fingers
> Left eye after surgery - 20/15

I am in my forties, and I wore glasses for more than twenty-five years. They were so heavy, they must have slid down my nose a thousand times a day.

As a teen, I missed playing sports for fear of breaking my glasses. Most importantly, myopia kept me from a career as a pilot.

I tried contact lenses, but I couldn't adjust to the hard lenses. I was allergic to the various solutions used with soft lenses, and the degree of my astigmatism could not be corrected.

Becoming a police officer introduced me to many new difficulties wearing glasses. Being in the cold, then entering a warm place, fogs the lenses. (This proved to be dangerous one night. I entered a house where a barricaded knife-wielding suspect had threatened to kill his hostage and himself. By blind luck, I was able to subdue and disarm the man without causing injury to anyone.) I was constantly fearful of losing my glasses while struggling with a person.

I had read about RK surgery, and when I saw Dr. Grandon, I almost had to be peeled off the ceiling when he told me I was an *ideal* candidate.

Even though your eye is open during surgery, you cannot see what is being done. There is no pain during the operation, and only temporary discomfort after it.

The next morning, I ran to the front window and removed the eye patch. I was speechless. I could see *everything clearly*!

DEBBIE, a volunteer fire fighter

>Right eye before surgery - 20/400
>Right eye after surgery - 20/25
>
>Left eye before surgery - 20400
>Left eye after surgery - 20/25

I'm sure many people will agree that wearing glasses or contact lenses is inconvenient, but also for me they proved to be a hindrance in some circumstances.

As a volunteer fire fighter, I found that having glasses get wet is not only an annoyance but dangerous. Concurrently, a fire fighter wearing contact lenses around extreme heat and smoke experiences painful burning and dryness in the eyes.

I'm very happy my perfect vision has been restored.

DARRYL, an engineer

>Right eye before surgery - 20/800
>Right eye after surgery - 20/20
>
>Left eye before surgery - 20/800
>Left eye after surgery - 20/20

My vision was correctable with contacts. I had worn them since the fourth grade, but it is nice to no longer need them or worry about taking care of them.

The preoperative jitters were worse than the LASIK surgery itself, and I experienced no pain after surgery. Best of all, I could see clearly the next morning.

FRED, a police officer

>Right eye before surgery - 20/400
>Right eye after surgery - 20/25
>
>Left eye before surgery - 20/200
>Left eye after surgery - 20/15

I started wearing glasses around the age of 10, and it didn't take long before I knew I didn't like them. I tried some hard contacts when I was 18. I was working at a gas station then. Several times, I would be working on a car up on the rack, and dirt would fall into my eyes. I'd instinctively rub my eyes, causing the contact to move toward the back of my eyes. I always had a devil of a time trying to fish them back around to the front.

When I was 21, I joined the Monroe (Michigan) Police Department. I found out that glasses and police work get along as well as cats and dogs. If your glasses fogged up, no one would stop in the middle of a fight while you wiped them off. I don't know how many pairs of glasses the city had to buy for me because I broke them on the job.

Since most larger police departments have vision requirements (usually 20/100 uncorrected), if I wanted to grow in my career, I knew I would have to improve my eyesight.

RK surgery was very easy. I had two procedures on my left eye and one on my right eye. (The second one on my left eye was necessary because I forgot to put in the eye drops as directed after the first operation).

During the healing process, it was very exciting being able to see without corrective lenses. I used to walk out on my front porch and look across at my neighbor's car. With my uncorrected right eye at 20/400, I could barely see the shape of the car. After two weeks after surgery, I could read the *license plate number*! (A very important part of a police officer's job.)

RACQUEL, a corporate travel planner

> Right eye before surgery - Count fingers at 6 feet
> Right eye after surgery - 20/20
>
> Left eye before surgery - Count fingers at 6 feet
> Left eye after surgery - 20/20

I always felt that my poor vision cheated me from doing things other people enjoyed doing. Swimming, riding the waves at a water park, and enjoying amusement rides.

I had been scheduled for RK surgery with Dr. Grandon, but after he told me about LASIK, we mutually agreed that it would be the best procedure for me. His self-confidence made me feel certain that he was the right one to perform the surgery.

I love my new vision, which, not so long ago, was just a dream.

KAISER, an award-winning artist

>Right eye before surgery - 20/400
>Right eye after surgery - 20/30
>
>Left eye before surgery - 20/400
>Left eye after surgery - 20/20

My vision got progressively worse from the fourth grade until the tenth grade when I got my first contacts. I had a difficult time in sports, because my glasses or contacts always got in the way.

Hard contacts scratched my corneas twice, so I switched to soft contacts. They didn't give me as much correction as I needed, but they were more comfortable to wear. Eventually, however, my eyes rejected them.

I'm very, very pleased with the results of RK surgery. Now I enjoy hassle-free living after years of being handicapped without my glasses or contact lenses.

ANNE, wife and mother

> Right eye before surgery - 20/600
> Right eye after surgery - 20/25
>
> Left eye before surgery - 20/600
> Left eye after surgery - 20/20

I wore contacts successfully for a number of years and pursued a variety of lifestyle activities. When my baby was born in early 1998, I switched to glasses. At that time, I went to the Eye Surgery Institute for an examination. I asked Dr. Grandon about corrective surgery.

I was so excited when he told me that I was a perfect candidate for LASIK surgery, and after conducting some research on my own about that procedure, I concluded it was the best one for me.

The decision proved to be right. I love the results!

NANCY B.

> Right eye before surgery - Count fingers at 6 feet
> Right eye after surgery - 20/40
>
> Left eye before surgery - Count fingers at 6 feet
> Left eye after surgery - 20/25

When I was six years old, I was fitted for my first pair of glasses. I remember flunking the eye exam in my first grade class; thus my visit to the doctor with *Diseases of the Eye* on his office door.

I was very sensitive about my thick lenses, which many people referred to as 'Coke bottle' bottoms. Being called *Four Eyes* was an almost daily occurrence.

For more than 21 years, I wore corrective lenses. Professionally and academically, people thought I was more intelligent because I wore glasses. It was socially that they were the biggest problem. It's hard to feel attractive with half-inch lenses on your face. Somehow my husband saw past them, but I feel much more confident in my appearance since RK surgery.

I was, at first, afraid of the RK procedure and its possible complications. On the morning of surgery, I was very scared. The surgery was painless and fast, however. I was uncomfortable for about three days afterward, at which time my vision came into focus.

Almost daily I am reminded how fortunate I have been, and it is a thrilling experience all over again.

SUSAN G.

>Right eye before surgery - 20/400
>Right eye after surgery - 20/20
>
>Left eye before surgery - 20/400
>Left eye after surgery - 20/20

I knew immediately that RK surgery was for me. I hated the way I looked in glasses, and contact lenses were painfully irritating to me.

I didn't expect to get 20/20 vision without any correction necessary. I thought I would still need glasses for driving, at least.

For me, it's been a miracle procedure. RK surgery was the answer to my vision problems, and the bothersome glare I experienced after surgery was minor compared to all the benefits of life without glasses.

Even though it's been several years since surgery, I still find myself wanting to push the eyeglasses that are no longer up there on my nose.

CHAPTER TWENTY-ONE
Questions & Answers

After reading this guide to refractive surgery, you may still have questions. Perhaps we can anticipate some of them.

Is radial keratotomy (RK) still investigational?

No. RK is no longer investigational. That tag was lifted some time ago by the American Academy of Ophthalmology. According to Dr. Ronald Schachar, executive secretary of the Kerato-Refractive Society in Denison, Texas, approximately 2,000 ophthalmologists were performing RK surgery in the United States, as of 1990. Today, many more are performing RK, because it is an accepted procedure and because it is being taught by many established RK surgeons like myself.

Schachar estimated that more than 500,000 radial keratotomy procedures have been performed in the United States as of early 1990. Today, that estimate has grown to more than a million.

Most significantly, in 1988, Waring, who directed the PERK Study, released the following statement:

> *A wealth of clinical and laboratory data have now defined a relative level of safety and effectiveness for the RK procedure.*

Is radial keratotomy a cosmetic procedure?

No. Cosmetic means a change in appearance. Radial keratotomy improves the function of two of the body's more vital organs: the eyes. Radial keratotomy enables nearsighted individuals to see better and, therefore, to improve many aspects of their lives.

Is radial keratotomy safe?

According to recent studies, radial keratotomy, on a statistical basis, is at least as safe as the long-term use of contact lenses. The number of serious complications has been extremely low. A more recent study indicates that radial keratotomy may be safer than even the use of eyeglasses.

Of course, if you are going to have radial keratotomy, you absolutely must go to a well-trained, very experienced surgeon, in my opinion, one who uses the American technique which, I believe, is safer than the Soviet technique.

Is the eye weaker after RK surgery?

In over 15,000 cases that I have performed, I have never encountered a situation where even severe trauma to the eye has opened the RK incisions, and I have performed RK on many police and security officers, as well as on fire fighters.

In fact, in severe trauma, it might be even safer to have an incision open and let the pressure out than have the *sclera* (back of the eye) tear, exposing the retina and vitreous.

Anecdotally, one police officer was in a severe accident in which he sustained very serious closed head injuries, but no trauma to the eyes, both of which had had RK surgery.

Animal experiments in the early years of RK showed that after healing, the eye is approximately as strong as it was before surgery. In approximately six months of the healing phase, the eye is in a weakened condition, however, so safety glasses should be worn in situations where the eye is at risk (certain sports and work conditions).

What kinds of questions can a prospective patient ask an ophthalmologist to determine if he/she has had experience in performing RK or AK?

I would ask the following questions:

> *How many years have you performed RK surgery?*
>
> *What techniques do you use?* [Again, in my opinion, the American RK technique is safer than the Soviet technique.]
>
> *How many cases have you performed?* [I personally would not undergo RK with an ophthalmologist who has performed fewer than 1,000 cases; or, at a minimum, the surgeon should not only have taken courses in RK surgery but also should have personally observed and studied with a respected RK expert.]
>
> *Do you perform RK surgery on a routine, weekly basis? Do you have a major commitment to refractive surgery (attend meetings, study new techniques, read articles, and so forth)?*

Are both eyes ever done at the same time in RK surgery?

Although some refractive surgeons perform surgery on both eyes at the same surgical appointment, I, and most of my fellow refractive surgeons, do not routinely do so. Everyone heals differently. We're dealing with a biological system, not just a theoretical situation. The nature of healing varies from one person to the next, so that no matter how sophisticated our computer software, how sharp our surgical knives, or how skilled our hands, we cannot completely predict the outcome of refractive surgery.

Performing surgery on the non-dominant eye first allows the surgeon to more accurately determine the parameters of surgery on the second eye. But, as with everything in life, rules are made to be broken. If someone is having simultaneous surgery to enhance moderate to low myopia or astigmatism following RK, with time and distance a problem, it is a major consideration. On the rare occasions when I do both eyes at the same surgical appointment, I always use a new set of instruments and a new drape for each eye. I prefer not to do it, but will do it for enhancements or touch-ups.

Can a person undergo RK surgery if she/he has astigmatism?

Yes. Surgery can correct both refractive problems at the same time. Also, astigmatism alone can be corrected by undergoing astigmatic keratotomy (AK).

How long do glare and fluctuating vision last after RK surgery?

Recent studies show that it takes the cornea three years or more to completely heal. Long before that, however, most people report that they experience little glare or fluctuating vision. In fact, very few of my patients have complained about glare or fluctuating vision after about one and a half years following surgery.

It is interesting to note that some people experience a small amount of fluctuating vision for many years after RK surgery, but usually it does not bother them, and sometimes it improves with time. For the rare individuals whose glare and fluctuating vision persist indefinitely, those problems usually can be taken care of by the new glare coating available for eyeglasses for night driving.

Interestingly, it has also been found that some people who have never had RK surgery experience some degrees of fluctuating vision.

Can a person be too myopic to get a complete result from RK surgery?

Yes. Today, in the United States, we feel that LASIK is preferred for patients with -6.0 diopters or more of myopia. While RK can be done for high myopes, newer technology yields better results with LASIK. Also, for very high myopes, phakic IOL surgery shows great promise for people over -15.0 D.

Will a person who has undergone refractive surgery be more likely to develop cataracts later in life?

No. In most cases, cataracts develop as part of a person's normal aging process. Neither radial keratotomy (RK), nor AK stops the aging of the eyes. If an RK patient develops cataracts later in life, he can be treated the same as if he had not had refractive surgery.

Knowing what power of lens implant to use for cataract surgery is very important. A great deal of research has been done lately with my brother, Dr. Gary Grandon. Again, it is important to go to a knowledgeable and experienced cataract surgeon who understands the parameters of determining the power of the lens implants.

Will a person who has had RK surgery need to wear reading glasses after he reaches the age of 40?

In most cases, when an individual reaches about 40, reading glasses become a necessity. The condition responsible for this need is aging, and the refractive problem is known as presbyopia, a form of farsightedness that is part of the person's normal aging process. Although there presently is a glimmer of hope that surgery can correct presbyopia, we are still a long way from having an accepted procedure.

There is a better range of vision (distance and near) in people who have had RK surgery than in those who have not. Some of my patients do not need reading glasses until they reach their early 50s. This situation is thought to be due to aspherosity of the cornea and multiple focal points after RK surgery.

What is the effect of RK surgery on the cornea?

At a meeting of the Kerato-Refractive Society in 1986, Dr. Fyodorov reported interesting news. He stated that the RK procedure rejuvenates the cornea. He explained that during the healing of the radial incisions, the cells lay down new collagen.

Pathological studies of corneas that had RK surgery have shown that the diameter of those collagen fibers is actually the same as that of embryonic (baby) collagen. "We're making the cornea younger and better," he announced. "If we could apply this knowledge to other body tissues, we could discover how to rejuvenate the entire body…not just corneas."

After RK surgery, how long will I have to take off work?

Some of my patients have gone back to work the day after surgery. The patch usually stays on for only an hour after surgery, but there may be sufficient discomfort when the anesthetic and medications wear off to warrant a full day of rest. If a person feels like going to work the next day, and the job poses no undue hazards to his eyes, he may feel free to do so. Safety glasses should be worn in any situation that warrants their use.

Some people experience quite a bit of light sensitivity and irritation, and may not be able to work for several days following RK surgery.

With the newer LASIK technique, there seems to be less pain and light sensitivity, and patients can now resume normal activities one or two days after surgery.

What are the long-term effects of RK surgery?

Radial keratotomy has been performed in Russia (formerly the Soviet Union) for 25 years and in the United States for more than 20 years. Most RK surgeons who perform large numbers of radial keratotomies report good stability and permanence of correction in their patients.

There is every reason for us to believe that these reports will continue to hold true. Corneal transplants, which require invasive eye surgery with through-and-through corneal incisions, have been performed for more than 75 years with complete healing and permanent correction.

If you have your nose shaped, as Fyodorov likes to say, it will not return to its former shape one day. The same holds true for the cornea. Reshaping the cornea, we believe, is also quite permanent.

How stable is RK? How stable is LASIK?

RK is very stable. The study we performed after three or four years showed that approximately 15% of RK patients became +1.0 D. more hyoperopic (farsighted). By the same token, 15% of our patients became more myopic. The great majority were quite stable. Other studies have shown a slight hyperopic shift, but in most cases it is not significant.

Occasionally a patient has more shifting, a situation that is often associated with people who rub their eyes a lot. After RK, it is imperative that one not rub his/her eyes. If the patient has allergies, he/she is instructed to use eyedrops to minimize the desire to rub the eyes.

In my own experience, people with larger hyperopic shifts were heavy eye rubbers.

LASIK seems to be very stable. There is very little fluctuation of vision throughout the day, which can sometimes be seen with RK, especially in higher myopes.

The reason we have confidence with the stability of LASIK is that the procedure's forerunner, keratomileusis, has been done since 1955. That is approximately 40 years with very good stability. Of course, all biological tissues change with time, so we cannot give a guarantee that in 10 or 20 years, there won't be any changes.

What is the highest degree of myopia that can be corrected with LASIK?

There are differing opinions about the highest degree of myopia that can be corrected with LASIK, but it is my opinion that the highest is -15D. Over that degree of myopia, with LASIK, there have been reports of glare with night driving.

There is much controversy at this time over this question. While there is evidence that LASIK can achieve correction up to -20D, there is consensus that over -15D, with LASIK, there is too much spherical aberration, loss of best corrected visual acuity, and difficulty with glare in night driving. The best results are -15D and under. The gap may eventually be filled with phakic IOLs or clear lens implants.

How long does the LASIK procedure take to perform?

The duration of the procedure depends on the degree of myopia, but, in general, it takes approximately six seconds for the keratome to make the flap, and the laser takes three minutes or less. From prep to finish, the entire procedure takes about 10 minutes. LASIK is a 10-minute miracle!

Can an overcorrected RK procedure be corrected with hyoperic LASIK?

Yes. In other countries with more experience with hyperopic LASIK, ophthalmologists have reported quite good results in correcting overcorrected RK. The Excimer Laser for hyperopia correction has now been approved by the FDA for use in the United States.

Can overcorrected myopia with LASIK be corrected?

Yes. Again, in the United States we have little experience with this. In other countries, they have done it successfully with LASIK, although there are far fewer overcorrections with LASIK than with RK.

Can anyone have LASIK?

No. Some individual who have deep-set eyes cannot undergo LASIK, because their eye openings are too small to accommodate the LASIK ring. Also, their corneas have to be healthy with no corneal problems.

What is your opinion of PRK (surface laser)?

In my opinion, this procedure is not very good (others may disagree). After the initial surface laser procedure, there is tremendous discomfort and pain; the patient must wear contact lenses for two to three days for epithelial healing; and, in some cases, corneal hazing may be permanent, necessitating the use of steroids for four to five months, which can also cause pressure problems in the eye and cataracts. There can also be late hazing three to four years after the procedure. Usually this problem is associated with people who live in sunny climates. Also, we do not know the long-term effect of the removal of Bowman's membrane.

For these reasons, I discourage patients from having surface laser surgery. I believe LASIK is a far superior procedure.

After LASIK, what restrictions, if any, are there?

We advise our LASIK patients to not swim for a week; and, especially, not rub their eyes for one to three days following the procedure. We provide a clear shield to cover the eye(s) for the first 24 hours to make it impossible for them to rub their eyes.

> No one can predict the future or where the technology goes from here for refractive surgery. The promise of the great parade of pioneers — Dr. Barraquer, Professor Fyodorov, and Dr. Bores — is now truly coming to fruition and is becoming a reality in ever safer procedures for the correction of myopia, hyperopia, and astigmatism with better results.
>
> The march of technology, given its relatively short time span, has been truly incredible. It has been an exciting period to be an ophthalmologist.

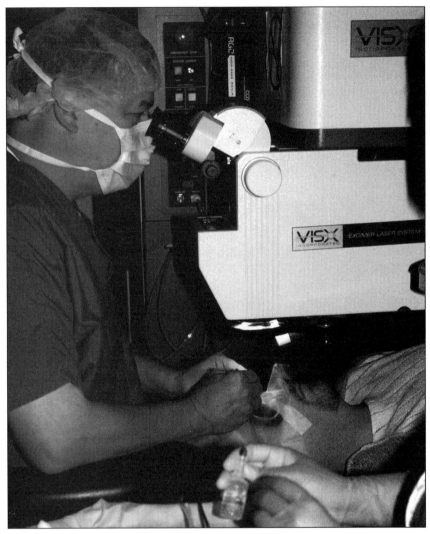
Dr. Stanley C. Grandon performing LASIK surgery.

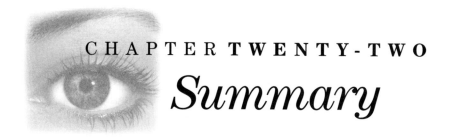

CHAPTER TWENTY-TWO
Summary

A former Chief of Ophthalmology at Kresge Eye Institute in Detroit, Dr. Robert Jampel, under whom I trained, once explained that there are two reasons why people go to a physician. One is for diagnosis, and the other is for the best treatment known at that time. Treatments are always changing, because technology is always changing. There is always controversy about what is the best treatment at any given time.

Refractive surgery is in its infancy, and the technology is rapidly changing. Treatment choices for the different refractive conditions are in a constant state of flux. The procedure thought to be the best one or two years ago may have already been replaced by newer technology. Therefore, when a patient sees an ophthalmologist, he should discuss the pros and cons of all possible procedures in order to arrive at the best decision.

At one time, RK had the advantage of being able to correct higher degrees of myopia, offering quicker rehabilitation of vision, less fluctuation of vision, and more long-term stability of vision. That advantage was offset by increasing experiences using LASIK. However, that was soon altered by the increasing possibility of serious complications with older flap makers and increasing possibility of loss of best corrected visual acuity (more so than with RK).

With the advances of the Hansatome Keratome, and newer ones in the state of development, however, LASIK has once again stepped onto center stage. The increased safety feature is one reason. If suction is lost during the flap making procedure, the Hansatome stops. The oscillating speed is now increased, too, and the precision of the Hansatome Keratome gives the surgeon considerably more confidence. With these newest advances, bilateral surgery is now possible; the results have exceeded our wildest expectations.

Nothing done by man is perfect. Every procedure has the potential for complications, either short or long term.

RK is an excellent procedure for -3D and under. Between -3D and -6D, either RK or LASIK works well; however, the price difference often becomes a deciding factor in the choice.

Most insurance companies do not pay for LASIK, whereas some pay for at least part of RK. In the future, maybe some will also pay for LASIK. LASIK is more expensive than RK, because the instruments are so much more expensive. The Hansatome Keratome costs $80,000 and backups are needed. The laser costs $500,000, and is expensive to maintain. The laser company charges a royalty fee of $250 per use. Also, expensive technicians are needed to keep the equipment operating well.

For someone who is -3D or less, the results of RK are excellent, at least with a highly experienced RK surgeon. Of the 16,000 cases I have performed, 98% received a result of 20/40 or better, with no serious complications and no significant loss of best corrected vision.

From -3D to -6D, approximately 90% achieve 20/40 or better with one procedure. With a touch-up, about 98% get 20/40 or better. These are good results. However, from -3D to -6D, the results with the newest LASIK technology seem to be even better.

With the older LASIK procedure, there were higher risks and more complications, such as problems with the flap, epithelial ingrowth with central scarring, and loss of best corrected vision. The newest advances in LASIK technology have greatly reduced these problems. For myopes over -6D, LASIK is now the preferred procedure. Although it is more expensive than RK, it is a safer option with fewer complications for -6D and up.

While RK gives quite good results, especially for -3D and under, LASIK — for the same degrees of myopia — may offer advantages, including the fact that surgery can be performed bilaterally, there is almost no pain, and there is quicker vision rehabilitation.

Dr. Grandon's Experience with LASIK

Being very conservative by nature, early I recognized the greatness of radial keratotomy (RK). I was impressed with the improved technology but also because the center of the cornea (2 to 3mm through which one sees) was not touched. Therefore, even if the result was not optimal, the patient, with glasses or contacts, could almost always see as well as he did before surgery and with very little loss of best corrected vision.

The problem with surface laser (PRK) and ALK is that the center of the cornea is violated. Any irregularity, hazing, or scarring of the center area of the cornea causes loss of best corrected visual acuity. Occasionally patients would get irregular astigmatism that could not be corrected with eyeglasses. Contact lenses would often alleviate the problem, but difficulty with contacts was often the reason the patient was having surgery in the first place.

SUMMARY

Technology marches on. With the advent of LASIK, technology took a giant leap forward. After the flap was made, instead of tissue being removed by another pass of the flapmaker, the laser, which is very accurate, was used to reshape the cornea beneath the flap. This is more accurate than the former oscillating blade technology, and results are much better.

However, results still weren't good enough. With the earlier keratome, there was occasional loss of pressure, a small flap might be made, or the flap might be button-holed (a hole or tear in the flap, leading to serious loss of best corrected visual acuity). Because of these occasional serious problems with earlier LASIK, because the surface laser had all sorts of problems with central scarring, pain, and because the results of RK were better, I felt it was not wise to perform LASIK.

Results of RK in my hands were better than with the results others were getting with the earlier LASIK technology, with far less chance of complication.

All this changed with the advent of the Hansatome Keratome, which seems to be the culmination of all previous flapmaker technology. Designed by Dr. Hansa and developed by Chiron, the Hansatome Keratome finally had the reliability and safety that made LASIK a quite safe and predictable procedure.

The Hansatome Keratome has many very high-tech safety features and is much simpler to use. Mistakes about depth of cut cannot be made. The Keratome will not run unless it is perfectly seated in the suction ring. If there is a loss of pressure, the Keratome stops immediately, practically eliminating the chance of irregular thinning or a small flap. Free flaps (flaps completely severed) become very rare. According to Chiron representatives, in 6,000 uses of the Hansatome

Keratome before general use, there were almost no significant flap problems.

Before I first performed LASIK, I was skeptical. With the first cases, I did just one eye. Everything went very smoothly. When I saw the patients the next day, I was truly amazed at how well they saw, how happy they were, and how little pain or discomfort they felt. The first two or three patients wanted their other eye done right away. They were the happiest patients I had ever seen.

When I first performed RK in 1982 on my own patients, the thing that impressed me was how happy they were after one or two weeks. These LASIK patients were incredibly happy the *next day* and exhibited very little of the postoperative symptoms associated with radial keratotomy, such as fluctuation, glare, light sensitivity, and quite a bit of discomfort. The LASIK patients saw very well with almost no discomfort or pain. I did their other eyes a week later and, uniformly, they were the happiest patients I had ever seen.

On the next group of patients, I did LASIK surgery on both eyes the same day. These patients were even happier than the first patients because now they saw beautifully with almost no discomfort or pain, almost no glare, and almost no fluctuation. I have never seen patients so happy this quickly.

I even had one patient who went to a movie the night of surgery, then walked around the city amazed at how well he could see a few hours after surgery.

Finally, the work of Dr. Barraquer, Professor Fyodorov, Dr. Bores, and other ophthalmologists like myself seems to be coming to fruition. This is truly a miracle!

My experience with LASIK continues to be very gratifying. This doesn't mean that all patients receive a postoperative result of 20/20 vision with LASIK. I am certain there will be occasional problems and reoperations. Still, I am truly a convert to the miracle of LASIK.

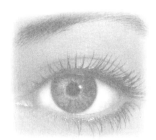

Glossary

Aniseikonia – difference in image size between a person's two eyes

Anisometropia – difference in power between a person's two eyes

Applanation tonometry – an ophthalmic examination given to determine eye pressure readings

Arcuate incision – a special "t" incision developed by Dr. Spencer Thornton for the correction of astigmatism

Astigmatism – a condition in which the curvature of the cornea is uneven, resulting in distant points in space being a blur on the retina

Automated Lamellar Keratoplasty – also known as ALK, a new procedure for the correction of refractive errors

Bowman's membrane – a membrane in the front of the eye that is vaporized during laser procedures

Clear lensectomy – lens extraction and IOL implant procedure

Clear zone (optical zone) – the central part of the cornea through which you see

Cornea – the clear front part (window) of the eyeball

Corneal flap – thin layer of corneal tissue

Corneal topography – an instrument in a computer-assisted videokeratometer which gives extremely accurate corneal readings and other corneal topography information

"Count fingers" – a vision test used for high myopes who cannot read an eye chart. The patient, instead, counts the number of fingers the examiner holds up at different distances

Diopter – a measure of myopia, hyperopia or astigmatism

Dosage dissection of the circumferential ligament of Cucute – the original Soviet name for the procedure now known as radial keratotomy

Enhancement – a touch-up or reoperation to achieve improved results in refractive surgery

Epikeratophakia – a surgical procedure for correcting high myopia that involves making a groove in the cornea and suturing in lathe-cut donor corneal tissue

Epithelium – the outer surface of the cornea

Excimer Laser – a "cold" laser used in a new procedure to carve the cornea into a new shape

Eye strain – an aching in the eye

Expert system – a computer program with which the surgeon consults to determine the precise surgical parameters he will use for an individual operation

Extasia – progressive corneal thinning

Eye chart measure – standard test to determine visual acuity. 20/40 means that at 20 feet (the first number), a person can read the smallest letter on an eye chart that a person with normal vision can read at 40 feet (the second number).

Fluctuating vision – different vision at different times of day. One of the expected postoperative conditions of RK surgery, fluctuating vision, which usually improves with time, can also occur in individuals who have not had RK surgery.

Fluorescein – a dye applied to the cornea, after it has been marked with a corneal marker, to enable the surgeon to more clearly see where the radial incisions will be made

4% Xylocaine – a topical anesthetic used in ophthalmic surgery

Hansatome Keratome – the most advanced, precise, and accurate keratome used for making corneal flap in LASIK procedure

Hexagon – the design of the procedure used to correct hyperopia (farsightedness). There are two hexagon patterns — the disconnected spiral hexagon and the overlapping hexagon.

Holmium Laser – a laser that is especially useful in treating glaucoma, and also for the correction of hyperopia and astigmatism

Hyperopia – commonly known as farsightedness; a condition which causes a point in space to focus behind the retina, making distant objects clear but near objects blurred

Intraocular lens – the lens placed inside the eye to correct vision; can be used for correction of myopia or hyperopia

Keratitis, ulcerative – an infection of the cornea which can be caused by extended use of contact lenses and which can be painful and destroy vision

Keratoconus – an abnormal shape of the cornea

Keratome – the flapmaker in LASIK and keratomileusis surgery

Keratomileusis – a procedure for correcting high myopia that involves removal of a thin layer of the cornea which is lathe-cut and sutured back onto the cornea

Knuckling – a non-surgical technique that helps under-corrected myopia patients achieve a better result

LASIK – a newer surgical procedure in which a flap is made on the cornea; the flap is flipped back; the corneal bed is lasered; and the hinged flap is replaced. [Acronym for Laser Assisted In Situ Keratomileusis]

Lid speculum – a tiny device used to hold open the upper and lower eyelids during ophthalmic surgery

Micrometer handle – the part of the diamond knife that enables the surgeon to adjust the blade to the desired depth of incision

Multiple Regression Analysis – a computer technique used to examine how well a particular combination of predictors fits known outcomes of RK surgery

Myopia – commonly known as nearsightedness; a condition which causes a point in space to focus in front of the retina, resulting in distant objects appearing blurred or fuzzy

Ophthalmic technician – an individual who is trained to perform eye examinations and assist ophthalmologists in surgery

Ophthalmologist – a medical doctor who can prescribe glasses, contact lenses, and medications, treat eye disorders, and perform eye surgery

Optic pachymeter – predecessor of the ultrasound pachymeter used to measure corneal thickness

Optical zone – also known as the clear zone, the central part of the cornea through which you see

Optician – a person trained to fit prescription glasses and contact lenses

Optometrist – an individual trained and licensed to test vision, prescribe glasses and contact lenses. An optometrist is *not* a medical doctor.

Orthokeratology – a technique of mechanically flattening the curvature of the cornea with a successive series of hard contact lenses. Used in cases of mild myopia.

PRK – photorefractive keratoplasty, the technical name for the procedure involving the Excimer Laser

Presbyopia – an aging condition in which the eye is unable to focus on near and far objects, resulting in a need for bifocals

Ptosis – droopy eyelid

Radial keratotomy – a surgical procedure in which radial incisions are made on the surface of the cornea to flatten the central part (clear zone), so that light will focus closer to the retina than it did before surgery. A permanent correction of myopia

Redeepening – a technique used to trace the initial radial incisions (in radial keratotomy) and make them deeper; for better correction in cases of high myopia

Retina – the layer of light-sensitive cells in the back of the eye

Sclera – back of the eye

Spherical equivalent – measurement of the closest spherical correction of hyperopia or myopia without astigmatism

Stroma – the middle of the cornea

Tangential incisions – certain incisions used to correct astigmatism in combination with radial incisions for the correction of myopia

Transverse incisions – also known as "flag" incisions; used to correct astigmatism

Trapezoidal keratotomy – also known as the Ruiz procedure, a surgical technique used to correct astigmatism

Ultrasound pachymetry – ultrasound equipment used to measure the thickness of the cornea

Visual acuity – a measure of how well a person can see under normal conditions

Visual axis – the axis of sharpest vision in the eye slightly medial to the center of the cornea

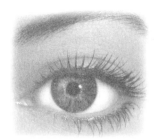

Index

A
Abrasion, corneal – 4
Accommodation – 1
AK – 83, 153, 154, 155
ALK – 28, 29, 81, 105, 113
American Academy of Ophthalmology – 41, 85, 86, 151
Analytical Radial Keratotomy Study Group (ARK) – 40, 130
Antibiotic eye drops – 79, 107
Applanation tonometry – 57
ARK – 41, 42, 55
Arrowsmith, Peter M.D. – 41, 130
Aspherosity – 77, 156
Astigmatic keratotomy (AK) – 20, 45, 51, 53, 60, 65, 66, 71, 77, 126
Astigmatism – 7, 18, 19, 20, 23, 29, 45, 48, 49, 52, 53, 56, 58, 60, 62, 65, 66, 72, 73, 77, 94, 99, 100, 101, 102, 104, 106, 115, 133, 141, 143, 154, 161
Astigmatism, induced – 48, 49, 50, 126
Astigmatism, irregular – 28, 100, 165
Automated Lamellar Keratoplasty (ALK) – 27, 100

B
Barraquer, Jose Ignacio, M.D. – 105, 117, 161, 167
Bifocals – 12, 16, 22, 62
Blue Cross/Blue Shield – 85, 86, 87, 88, 89
Bores, Leo, M.D. – 33, 34, 36, 37, 39, 40, 44, 75, 130, 161, 167
Bowman's membrane – 28, 99, 101, 160

C
Cafferty, Michael S. – 87
Cataracts – 6, 33, 67, 107, 122, 123, 125, 126, 127, 155, 160
Chiron – 166
Clear zone – 33, 40, 72, 74, 84, 131
Clear lensectomy – 125, 126

Clear lens extraction – 126, 127
Clear lens implant – 18, 159
Contact lenses – 5, 6, 7, 10, 12, 16, 17, 18, 19, 21, 23, 24, 34, 57, 58, 63, 66, 76, 80, 81, 97, 108, 113, 121, 132, 143, 144, 145, 146, 147, 148, 152, 160, 165
Contact lenses, bifocal – 24
Contact lenses, extended wear – 24, 25, 26
Contact lenses, gas permeable – 23, 24
Contact Lens Institute – 26
Cornea – 1, 2, 3, 4, 7, 11, 12, 19, 25, 26, 27, 28, 29, 32, 33, 38, 46, 47, 51, 61, 66, 71, 74, 75, 76, 77, 83, 92, 93, 95, 99, 100, 102, 105, 113, 114, 117, 118, 123, 127, 147, 154, 156, 158, 160, 165
Corneal curvature – 131
Corneal flap – 28, 66, 104, 105, 107, 109, 110, 111, 112, 114, 118, 119, 120, 159, 165, 166
Corneal marker -73
Corneal thinning – 68, 123
Corneal topography – 6, 7, 58
Corneal ulcer – 24, 25, 68
"Count fingers" test – 13
Cowden, John W. M.D. – 87
Crystalline lens – 2

D

Decentration – 68, 119
Diamond knife – 37, 39, 58, 74, 75, 101
Dietz, Michael M.D. – 41, 130
Diopter – 12, 13, 19, 28, 33, 38, 40, 43, 48, 55, 56, 60, 75, 76, 77, 93, 97, 103, 106, 116, 123, 126, 132, 155, 159
Ditzen, Klaus M.D. – 117
Dominant eye – 59, 126
Double vision – 63, 67

E

Ellipitical clear zone – 77
Enhancement – 56, 57, 76, 82, 112, 154
Endothelial cell loss – 68, 124
Epikeratophakia – 28
Epithelial downgrowth – 120
Epithelial healing defects – 68
Epithelial ingrowth – 119, 165

Epithelial irregularity – 106
Epithelium – 25, 95, 99, 113
Excimer Laser – 28, 66, 68, 91, 93, 94, 97, 98, 100, 101, 102, 103, 104, 106
Expert system – 130, 131, 135, 137, 140
Extasia – 68
Eyeglasses – 5, 6, 9, 10, 15, 16, 18, 19, 21, 22, 23, 29, 32, 59, 62, 63, 66, 76, 80, 82, 97, 108, 113, 116, 121, 122, 126, 132, 143, 144, 145, 146, 147, 148, 149, 150, 152, 155, 156, 165
Eye strain – 17
Eye Surgery Institute – 55, 61, 71, 80, 132, 134, 137, 148

F

Farsightedness – 15, 16, 17, 18, 19, 27, 45, 48, 50, 66, 93, 94, 106, 115, 117, 123, 156
Fluctuating vision – 44, 48, 62, 67, 80, 83, 97, 114, 115, 154, 155, 163, 167
Food & Drug Administration (FDA) – 23, 24, 25, 26, 28, 69, 93, 99, 101, 124, 127
Fyodorov, Svyatoslav, M.D. – 31, 32, 33, 34, 36, 37, 38, 39, 40, 44, 75, 81, 156, 158, 161, 167

G

Glare – 28, 48, 58, 62, 68, 79, 83, 97, 114, 154, 155, 159, 167
Glaucoma – 6, 67, 98, 100
Glaucoma, pupillary block – 127
Grady, Frank, M.D. – 130
Grandon, Gary M. Ph.D. – 57, 129, 131, 155

H

Hansatome Keratome – 118, 119, 120, 164, 166
Haze, corneal – 28, 67, 96, 97, 99, 100, 102, 103, 104, 114, 119, 160
Hemorrhage – 68
Hexagon, connected – 46, 48
Hexagon, disconnected – 46, 47
Hexagon, disconnected spiral – 47, 48, 49, 50
Hexagonal keratotomy (HK) – 16, 18, 45, 47, 49, 51
Hirschman, Henry M.D – 121
Holmium Laser – 91, 98, 101
Homoatropine – 118
Hyperopia – 15, 16, 17, 18, 20, 27, 46, 49, 51, 93, 98, 99, 100, 101, 104, 106, 117, 119, 120, 125, 126, 127, 161
Hyperopic LASIK – 51, 117, 120, 159
Hyperopic shifting – 43, 158

I

Implant, intraocular lens – 33, 106, 121, 125
Implants, clear lens – 18, 159
Incisions, arcuate – 53, 66, 74
Incisions, flag – 48, 49, 51, 52, 56, 77, 141
Incisions, "t" – 48, 49, 51, 53, 66, 74, 77
Incisions, transverse – 56
Induced astigmatism – 48, 49, 50, 126
Informed consent – 57, 61, 64, 65, 67, 68, 69, 83
Intraocular lens – 122, 126, 127
Intraocular pressure – 104, 118, 131, 160
Iris – 2, 3, 123
Irregular astigmatism – 28, 100, 165
Irregular thinning – 166

J

Jampel, Robert M.D. – 163

K

Katzen, Leeds M.D. – 37
Kera-Stat – 130, 137, 138, 139, 140, 141
Keratoconus – 7, 108
Keratectomy – 114
Keratome – 29, 105, 107, 109, 110, 112, 114, 159, 166
Keratometer – 19
Keratometry – 57
Keratomileusis – 27, 28, 100, 105, 117, 158
Kerato-Refractive Society – 151, 156
Knuckling – 82
KOI – 39
Kremer, Fred M.D. – 38, 130
Kresge Eye Institute – 37, 87, 163

L

Lamellar corneal transplant – 68
LASIK – 7, 18, 20, 28, 43, 44, 56, 60, 66, 67, 68, 69, 77, 81, 97, 100, 104, 105, 106, 107, 109, 111, 112, 113, 114, 115, 116, 119, 120, 125, 145, 147, 148, 155, 158, 159, 160, 163, 164, 165, 166, 167, 168
Lens – 1, 16, 17, 18, 125, 127
Lens extraction – 122, 125
Lens replacement – 122
Lid speculum – 72, 95, 110, 118
Light sensitivity – 28, 67, 157, 167

M

Marks, Ronald G., Ph.D. – 41
Mendez, Antonio M.D. – 45, 46, 47
Michigan Ophthalmology Society – 85, 86, 87, 88
Microkeratome – 68, 117, 118, 119
Monovision – 126
Multiple Regression Analysis – 136
Myers, William D. M.D. – 37, 38
Myopia – 1, 11, 12, 13, 15, 20, 21, 22, 23, 26, 27, 28, 32, 33, 35, 40, 42, 43, 44, 51, 52, 55, 56, 58, 59, 60, 61, 63, 72, 75, 76, 77, 85, 93, 97, 99, 100, 102, 103, 104, 106, 116, 117, 123, 125, 126, 127, 132, 133, 134, 136, 137, 138, 143, 154, 155, 159, 160, 161, 163, 165

N

National Eye Institute – 43
National Institute of Health – 41
Nearsightedness – 10, 11, 19, 20, 64, 66, 67, 93, 94, 96, 97, 101, 113, 115, 123
Nomograms – 136
non-dominant eye – 59, 126, 154

O

Opacification, corneal – 103
Ophthalmic technician – 6, 12
Ophthalmic technologist – 71
Ophthalmologist – 5, 6, 12, 18, 24, 26, 33, 35, 42, 45, 50, 55, 57, 59, 63, 64, 65, 104, 129, 151, 153, 159, 161, 163
Optic center – 118
Optic nerves – 1
Optical zone – 33, 47, 74, 100
Optical zone marker – 95
Optician – 5
Optometrist – 5, 12
Orbit – 1, 4
Orthokeratology – 21, 26, 27
Overcorrection – 59, 63, 68, 81, 102, 136, 159, 160

P

Periphery – 76
PERK – 43, 151
Phacoemulsification – 121
Phakic IOL – 18, 76, 123, 124, 155, 159

Photoablation – 118
Photorefractive keratoplasty (PRK) – 28, 94, 97
Predictability software – 37, 40, 129
Prediction equations – 136
Presbyopia – 16, 17, 67, 156
PRK – 98, 102, 103, 104, 107, 114, 119, 125, 160, 165
Prospective Evaluation of Radial Keratotomy (PERK) – 42
Ptosis – 68
Pupil –1, 2, 115, 124
pupillary block glaucoma – 127

Q

R

Radial keratotomy (RK) – 7, 29, 31, 32, 33, 34, 35, 36, 37, 38, 40, 41, 42, 43, 44, 45, 47, 48, 55, 56, 59, 61, 62, 64, 65, 71, 72, 73, 74, 75, 76, 77, 79, 81, 82, 83, 84, 85, 86, 87, 88, 89, 95, 100, 101, 102, 107, 120, 126, 127, 129, 130, 131, 133, 134, 135, 136, 139, 140, 141, 142, 144, 146, 147, 149, 150, 151, 152, 153, 154, 155, 156, 157, 158, 163, 164, 165, 166, 167
Redeepening – 56, 76, 84
Regression toward the mean – 136, 137
Retina – 1, 2, 11, 12, 15, 17, 18, 19, 152
Retinal degeneration – 67
Retinal detachment – 6, 67, 68
Ruiz, Luis M.D. – 51, 52, 77, 105

S

Sanders, Donald – 41, 47
Sawelson, Harold M.D. – 41
Scarring –28, 29, 50, 67, 100, 114, 119, 165, 166
Schachar, Ronald M.D – 17, 40, 151
Sclera – 1, 3, 152
Shepard, Dennis, M.D. – 38, 52
Shifting, hyperopic – 43
Silicone lenses – 23
Slit lamp – 6, 98, 99, 111
Spherical aberration – 159
Spherical equivalent – 132, 133, 139
Spigelman, Alan M.D. – 91, 105
Statistical analysis – 130, 137
Statistical software – 131
Steroids – 67, 82, 96, 98, 102, 104, 107, 118

Stroma – 28
Suction ring – 105, 110, 114, 118, 119, 166
Sunrise Holmium Laser – 98
surface ablation – 28
surface laser (PRK) – 29, 107, 119, 160, 165
swelling, corneal – 68

T
"t" incisions – 48, 49, 51, 53, 66, 74, 77
Thornton, Spencer M.D. – 53, 130
Topical anesthetic – 66, 72, 83, 94, 98, 118
Touch-up – 56, 57, 82, 84, 154, 164
Transverse incisions – 56
Trapezoidal keratotomy – 51, 77

U
Ulcerative keratitis – 25
Ultrasound A-Scan – 7
ultrasound pachymeter – 7, 37, 38, 58
undercorrection – 57, 63, 68, 82

V
Videokeratometer – 6, 58
Vision, double – 63, 67
Visual acuity – 28, 29, 40, 57, 81, 84, 93, 96, 97, 100, 101, 102, 103, 104, 118, 119, 131, 132, 133, 159, 163
Visual axis – 29, 75, 95, 99, 100, 101, 114, 124
VISX STAR Excimer Laser – 91, 92, 109

W
Waring, George III M.D. – 42, 107, 151
Williams, Dennis L M.D. – 125
Wilson, Louis MD – 25

X
Xylocaine – 72

Y
YAG laser – 100
Young, Frank E. M.D. – 26

Z